The
Greener
Side
of the FENCE

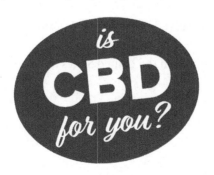

CATHERINE CATTARELLO AND ERIC SWEATT

CONTENTS

PART THREE

Work with Your Doctor!; Cytochrome P450 Enzymes;
Bioavailability; Potency or Concentration; Universal Laws; CBD
and Metabolism; Closing thoughts

Establish Your CBD Goals; Start Low and Go Slow; Micro-dosing;
Options for Taking CBD; Getting Off Traditional/Pharmaceutical
Medication(s); Closing Thoughts

PART FOUR

Who is causing all the commotion?; Big Pharma enters the picture;
What about legalization?; Guidelines, anyone?; What does the
research say?; Headline News!; Where do we go from here?;
Cultivation; Extraction; Processing and refining; Isolation of
valuable cannabinoids; Closing Thoughts

Distinguishing between Cannabis Medicine and Adult Recreational
Marijuana; A Clear Role for Pharmacists; What about Doctors?;
What does the research show?; Where do we go from here?;
Will marketing CBD change?; A post-pandemic CBD market?;
Sustainability in the Cannabis Industry; Closing thoughts Chapter 9

DISCLAIMER

AS HARD AS WE'VE WORKED to provide accurate information, we realize there is a possibility of human error, or changes to industry standards as the science continues to advance. Neither the authors, nor the publishers, nor any other party involved in the preparation or publication of this work, warrants the information included here is, in every respect, accurate or complete. They are not responsible for any errors or omissions, or for the results obtained from using this information. *Readers are encouraged to confirm the information contained in the book with other sources.* The Food and Drug Administration has not evaluated any of the statements made in this book. This information is intended to be educational only; it is not intended to diagnose, treat, cure, or prevent any disease.

INTRODUCTION

OUR HOPE FOR THIS BOOK has always been to provide enough information about CBD that anyone who is "on the fence" about trying it will be able to make an informed decision for themself. The title of the book, *The Greener Side of the Fence*, reflects this priority. As you proceed through the book, you'll recognize we believe strongly in interconnectedness, and in homeostasis, or a state of balance. We think a truly healthy lifestyle requires balance between all the interconnected elements of life. Unfortunately, life in the current era leaves most of us feeling seriously out of balance, which takes a toll on most people's health in one way or another.

Healthy people describe health as more than a goal or a dream. Health, they say, is a lifestyle. Sure, living a healthy lifestyle helps prevent chronic disease and long-term illness, but there is so much involved that making healthy choices isn't always an easy, straight forward decision. For example, how do you know if drinking coffee is good for you or not? Plenty of people say it is, and plenty others disagree. So, whom do you believe? What about eating gluten-free? Are meat and dairy products essential for a well-balanced diet, or is a plant-based diet better? These and many, many other questions like them often leave people feeling confused and overwhelmed about healthy nutrition. And nutrition is just one part of the complicated equation that adds up to a healthy lifestyle.

In the current era, living a healthy lifestyle seems more difficult than ever. The COVID-19 pandemic has certainly taken its toll on everyone. As we prepare to go to press, we've been dealing with the pandemic for two full years. We've gotten used to wearing masks, socially distancing, eating at home. Sadly, the death toll from COVID-19 continues, despite our collective best efforts. Additionally, substance abuse and addiction are spiraling out of control, despite decades of efforts to end this nightmare. Suicide rates are higher than ever, again despite decades of efforts to prevent this tragedy. Every single day the news is laden with reports of people being shot and killed, leaving all of us with a heightened awareness of just how vulnerable we really are. Politics are increasingly divisive, people are protesting in the streets, public officials are proving themselves considerably less than upright citizens. We are all struggling to make sense of this world, and to figure out whom we can trust. Can we possibly find balance amidst all of this?

Then, when we factor in each person's family issues, health challenges, and financial burdens, we realize finding a healthy balance definitely seems more difficult than ever. Not only do we all have confusion and frustration around nutrition, but managing our mental health in these difficult times has become a pretty immense challenge. And unfortunately, the incidence of physical health challenges increases proportionately to the incidence of mental health challenges. Often enough, we feel like *everything* is out of balance.

What does any of this have to do with CBD oil? A lot, actually. For one thing, CBD has proven to be an effective aid for various mental health challenges, especially depression and anxiety. But the main reason is because we believe people who are actively pursuing an overall healthy lifestyle will be happier with their results from taking CBD than those who are looking for a quick fix to whatever is ailing them.

We would love to think everyone who reads this book will have a positive experience with CBD and a good outcome from using it. Although CBD is definitely not a cure-all, it has helped multitudes of people living with multitudes of health challenges, and you could be among them. We certainly hope so! And you will probably get the best result from a CBD regimen if it is part of a holistic plan to live a healthy lifestyle. People who are paying attention to their diet, exercising within their abilities, regularly getting a good night's sleep, abstaining from cigarettes, drinking alcohol in moderation, and following their doctors' advice about taking medications, are considerably more likely to be pleased with the results of their CBD therapy than those who are not.

The journey of writing this book has taken three years. During this time, we have checked untold numbers of sources, especially those considered legitimate in the industry and those seen as reliable and thorough. We've conducted hours and hours and hours of research about CBD; a list of our sources is included at the back of the book. These are the sources we found valuable, but we strongly encourage readers to verify the information contained in the book with these and other credible sources.

Along the way, we've seen advances in research so that some parts of the book had to be rewritten to reflect the most up-to-date information. We've seen laws change, and with them, the general attitude of the population, as a whole, is shifting toward acceptance of and belief in the legitimacy of Cannabis Medicine. The industry is changing quicky.

When I started my research about CBD, trying to decide for myself whether it was something I wanted to try, I was shocked to find out how difficult it was to sort through the vast amount of data, then analyze and interpret the research. As a woman living with multiple sclerosis, a progressive neurologic disorder, I wanted to know if CBD might help ease some of my symptoms. I had heard stories about CBD not only easing people's symptoms, but in some cases actually halting people's symptoms, and in other cases actually stopping the disease progression. These miraculous possibilities are the exact opposite of what traditional western medicine typically offers people living with MS.

By comparison, the possibilities associated with CBD sounded too good to be true. I felt a tentative combination of hope and skepticism, but I was curious enough about getting the "real scoop" to continue my research. Often enough, following the clues was not straight forward, and it wasn't easy. Complicating the picture, as I dove into the research, I found a tremendous amount of conflicting information that left me wondering which was the right answer and whom should I believe? Determined to get to the root of things, I jumped in with both feet, turned over every stone, followed the clues, addressed difficult questions to as many experts as I could find.

One of those experts was Eric, who has been working in the industry for many years. Eric is the owner/director of *Medical Cannabis Outreach* in Illinois, plus a chain of CBD stores in Colorado, and most recently, owner of a line of CBD products, *Glacier Pure CBD*. Having worked with hundreds of people who benefited from a CBD regimen without any idea what CBD is or how/why it works, Eric was frustrated about the difficulty of getting valid information into people's hands. He had been approached by several doctors asking him for advice about working with their patients who were interested in CBD. Clearly, doctors, as well as consumers, need access to information about CBD.

As we shared our frustrations about the challenges of finding legitimate information about CBD and making it available to people who could use it, we decided to work together. We pooled our knowledge, wisdom, experience, and research skills together to compile the information we wished was more easily available. This book is the outcome of those efforts.

The book is organized so that Part One has general information and some history about CBD and Cannabis Medicine. We identified areas where information was either extremely difficult to find or was so conflicting it was almost impossible to sort through, or in some cases where false rumors were incorrectly being considered true. Referring to these as "black holes" of information, we point out the origin of the controversy and where the true answers lie. Some of these points continue being muddied by inconsistencies at the federal level. Though we point out these paradoxes, we are not interested in painting a negative picture of the federal government or any of its agencies and/or departments. We are only interested in clearing the muck that continues clouding legitimate information about CBD.

Part Two is about the science of how and why CBD works. We present detailed information about the synergy at play between the various chemical elements of cannabis plants and explain that human bodies produce chemical compounds remarkably similar to those found in cannabis plants. We explain in great detail how human bodies host an endocannabinoid system whose purpose is to maintain homeostasis throughout the body. And we explain, at least a little bit, about how it works and the medicinal potential this system represents. This section is loaded with some awfully dense science – enough that some readers might not really appreciate the material. So, please skip directly to Chapter 5 if the science behind CBD isn't particularly interesting to you.

Part Three discusses considerations each person will need to make once they've decided to get started with CBD. We adamantly encourage everyone to work with your doctor, though there is a possibility you might need to help your doctor become informed about Cannabis Medicine. We encourage everyone to establish goals you hope to accomplish with your CBD therapy, and we address how to get started taking CBD.

Finally, in Part Four we explore a bit about what the future may hold for the CBD industry and CBD consumers. The industry seems poised to continue changing quickly. There are currently proposals for marijuana legalization at the federal level before Congress, which will impact the CBD industry if passed. At the same time, many states continue evolving their policies and mandates around CBD. And, regardless of the politics surrounding CBD, research is advancing at a pretty fast pace. We explore some of the areas likely to be in line for changes as the research continues. We try to analyze how likely it is that the FDA will develop guidelines for the CBD industry, and try to explore the question of whether the FDA will approve additional cannabinoid-based medications, now that Epidiolex has opened that door. We examine some of the ways CBD and traditional medicine are already working together, and explore areas that appear ripe for advancements down this path. Finally, in the last chapters we state our personal hopes and expectations for the industry moving forward.

Throughout the book are stories of brave trailblazers who jumped off the fence and are helping lead the way, or blazing the trail, with CBD as medicine. You will read about people whose lives have been changed by their interest in and willingness to use CBD as medicine, even when most people did not consider it a smart strategy, especially most doctors. Many of these trailblazers have had the privilege of working with doctors who did not discourage them from using CBD, but none of them has been lucky enough to find a doctor who could help guide them down the trail of using CBD, especially when they wanted to blend it with traditional western medicine.

We encourage all doctors to step up to the plate and recognize Cannabis Medicine for the tremendous potential it offers patients. There is no reason for doctors to remain in the dark about the burgeoning field of Cannabis Medicine. We believe it would serve patients well for doctors to recognize how CBD can represent options for their patients who, often enough, are not satisfied with the limited options traditional western medicine makes available to them. We offer our sincere thanks and appreciation to all the trailblazers who have shared their CBD stories with us. We've also included a chapter written by a trailblazing doctor, and we thank her for her contribution to this book, and encourage her to share her wisdom and knowledge generously – both with her patients, and especially with her colleagues.

Around the world, people have been using cannabis as medicine for thousands of years. Only in relatively recent times has it been considered something other than medicinal, and the shift was driven by politics, not medicine. As the pendulum swings, people are again recognizing the tremendous medicinal potential within cannabis plants, and many people, especially CBD enthusiasts, are enjoying this fresh perspective. Long-standing limitations and restrictions on research are beginning to ease, opening the doors to untold further uses for this promising compound. Hemp and hemp-derived products are essentially legal at the federal level now, and most states have legal medical marijuana programs. These are clear indicators the times are changing, and people -- even government officials -- are recognizing the health benefits the amazing cannabis plant can offer.

The political landscape is also changing quickly, and it is more friendly toward cannabis now than it has been at any other time in recent history. Many people are anticipating marijuana will be legalized at the federal level sometime soon. Time will tell how that plays out, but in the meantime, hemp-derived products are essentially legal at the federal level and hemp-derived CBD continues helping multitudes of people living with multitudes of health challenges.

Wherever you are on your wellness journey, we believe information is power. Hopefully you will find the answers to your questions about CBD on the pages of this book. Whether you decide to use CBD or not to, you can now make your choice based on credible information. We wish you the best on your journey of healthy living.

PART
One

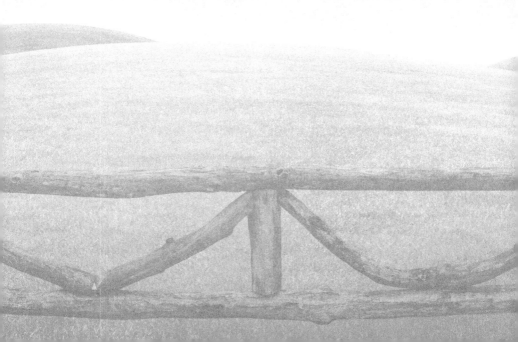

"*What we could consider magic, may just be science that we don't understand yet.*"

—PATRICIA ROBIN WOODRUFF

Chapter

1

CBD HAS STORMED OUT OF THE CLOSET and onto the shelves at just about every store in town, it seems. This compound has been called everything from a cure-all to modern-day snake-oil, but it is definitely presenting its face on every-other corner and in places that used to seem pretty unlikely. One thing is certain, though; CBD and its barrage of products are here to stay. Now one of the fastest growing industries in America and around the globe, it's hard to imagine there are still people who haven't heard of CBD. But there are plenty of people who don't really know anything about it, or who have been told something about it that doesn't seem right, or who doubt its true benefits. Choosing to err on the side of caution rather than risk becoming a victim of misinformation, many people have automatically decided not to try CBD.

Plenty of people are using CBD products, though. Stories about the record-breaking revenue from CBD products are reported regularly, indicating sales of CBD will continue to grow at an extraordinary pace. A 2019 study from *The Hemp Business Journal*, one of the most highly respected sources in the industry, found the field of CBD products will continue to grow at an astonishing rate.[1] The study predicted a new player entering the arena, the pharmaceutical industry, and that it will become the leader. This prediction was based on the fact that huge pharmaceutical companies carry clout and influence that small, independent CBD companies don't, including the ability to compel product testing and clinical trials from federal agencies like the Food and Drug Administration (FDA). They also have strong lobbying power with the Drug Enforcement Agency (DEA).

Like all robust industries, CBD is not without its critics. Frankly, CBD has a dark history in the United States. Clouded by years of misinformation, CBD's reputation has been largely driven by cannabis' status as a Schedule 1 Controlled Substance since the 70s and the launch of the US government's infamous *War on Drugs*. In the United States, CBD is generally produced from hemp, which has been, until very recently, lumped into a broad category with its sister, marijuana.

IS CBD MARIJUANA?

One of the "black holes" confounding people is whether or not CBD is a marijuana product? Knowing marijuana has been, and is still, classified as a Schedule 1 Controlled Substance leaves plenty of people unwilling to consider trying CBD. They don't know or understand that hemp-derived CBD is not the same product as marijuana-derived CBD, and it is essentially legal in all 50 states and US territories, as long as the hemp was grown by a licensed farmer in compliance with all state and federal laws.

The report in *The Hemp Business Journal* stated, "Competition between hemp-derived and marijuana-derived companies are expected to increase, with dozens of companies operating in both channels." It went on to state marijuana-derived CBD products were holding a slight edge at the time (2019), but it was quickly slipping to sales of hemp-derived products. The authors of the report went on to predict dispensaries, smoke shops, and health boutiques would probably lose their hold on the market. The industry is changing quickly.

WHAT, EXACTLY, IS CBD?

CBD is an acronym for Cannabidiol, a naturally occurring chemical compound found in the resinous flowers and other parts of Cannabis, a plant whose medicinal heritage has been strong for thousands of years. CBD is one of more than a hundred cannabinoids, or chemical compounds found in cannabis plants, that make up its therapeutic profile. CBD is safe for human consumption, even in very high doses, and it is non-addictive.

We've read a number of references that insist CBD is not psychoactive, but we wholeheartedly disagree. We understand people are making the point that, unlike THC, another cannabinoid in cannabis plants, CBD will not cause the "high" associated with marijuana. CBD does not have the intoxicating effect of THC and it does not cause cognitive alterations or withdrawal effects.

However, a chemical is considered psychoactive when it acts primarily on the central nervous system and alters brain function, resulting in temporary changes in perception, mood, consciousness, or behavior. CBD crosses the blood-brain barrier and directly affects the central nervous system, causing changes in mood and perception; it has been shown to have moderating effects on anxiety, psychosis, depression, pain, appetite, memory, seizures, and other brain activity. CBD works in tandem with THC and other canna-binoids that act on the central nervous system, but it does not result in euphoria or intoxication. We prefer to say CBD is non-intoxicating, but it is absolutely psychoactive. To say CBD is non-psychoactive is not correct, and it is misleading.

The purpose of this book is to shine a little light into some of the black holes of inconsistencies and misinformation about CBD. One of these dark areas is the relationship between hemp, cannabis, and marijuana. These terms are often used interchangeably, but they are actually not the same. According to the International Association for Plant Taxonomy, *"Both hemp(varieties) and marijuana (varieties) are of the same genus, Cannabis, and the same species, Cannabis Sativa."*[2] Another way of saying this might be, in this particular plant family, Cannabis is the grandparent, Cannabis Sativa is the parent, Hemp and Marijuana are offspring siblings, but they are not identical twins.

The words "cannabis" and "marijuana" are often used back and forth without distinction, perpetuating the confusion about their meanings. But the word "cannabis" refers to the entire genus of plants, including both hemp and marijuana. The word "marijuana" distinguishes between cannabis that is hemp and cannabis that isn't.

In the US, the difference between hemp and marijuana is determined by the amount of delta-9-tetrahydrocannabinol (THC) in any specific plant. THC is another cannabinoid; it is the chemical compound that causes the psychoactive high associated with marijuana. In the US, any cannabis plant containing more than 0.3% THC is marijuana, and cannabis plants with 0.3% or less of THC are hemp. In many other countries, the established difference between hemp and marijuana is 0.2% THC. Both in the US and in other countries, the trace amounts of THC in hemp are not enough to cause the psychoactive high associated with marijuana, which is one reason hemp-derived CBD products are so popular. Although hemp and marijuana are both classified as cannabis, there are a number of important differences between them, including the fact that hemp is not used as a recreational drug, nor could it be.[3]

We've seen several sources use these words incorrectly, and at least one explained they don't like to use the word "marijuana" because it has racial connotations, so they simply use the word "cannabis" instead. Which might be okay if they weren't writing about the differences between hemp and that other plant.

By racial connotations, we're pretty sure they are referring to the fact that the number and ratio of people who are either serving, or have served, time on marijuana charges are disproportionately people of color. Sadly, we knowingly agree the tangled web of the criminal justice system holds some people in its sticky strands with a much tighter fist than others. However, the purpose of this book is to cut through the confusion surrounding hemp-derived CBD, so we will use the scientifically correct names of the plants throughout the book. Just as a rose is a rose, marijuana is marijuana.[4]

A STORIED PAST?

The United States' decades-long prohibition of cannabis was founded on racism and bigotry. President Nixon's *War on Drugs* and its criminalization of cannabis are intrinsically muddled into the dirty water of systemic forces that have marginalized and antagonized people of color in the US since time immemorial. A department of the federal government that was the predecessor of the DEA, the Federal Bureau of Narcotics (FBN), was opened in 1930 as an agency of the US Department of the Treasury. The FBN was created to consolidate the functions of the Federal Narcotics Control Board and the Narcotics Division.

Founding commissioner of the FBN, Harry Anslinger, was a notorious bigot known for spewing utterly disparaging comments about people of color and indiscriminately associating them with illegal drugs. Under his prevailing attitude of hatred and inequality, congress passed the Marihuana Tax Act in 1937, effectively criminalizing cannabis. Because the laws prohibiting cannabis bundled hemp into the same package with its sister marijuana, hemp and hemp-derived products like CBD were also outlawed. In the 1950s, federal laws established mandatory sentences for drug-related offenses. Then, during the 60s, reports commissioned by both President Kennedy and President Johnson found marijuana was not a gateway drug and it would not provoke acts of violence. In 1972, the bipartisan Shafer Commission, appointed by President Nixon at the direction of Congress, determined personal use of marijuana should be decriminalized. Nixon rejected the recommendation.[5]

To this day, people of color in the US are arrested for drug offenses, including marijuana charges, at rates dramatically higher than white people. According to *The Drug Policy Alliance*:

- People of color experience discrimination at every stage of the criminal justice system and are more likely to be stopped, searched, arrested, convicted, harshly sentenced, and saddled with a lifelong criminal record. This is particularly the case for drug law violations.
- Nearly 80% of people in federal prisons and almost 60% of people in state prisons for drug offenses are black or Latino.
- Prosecutors are twice as likely to pursue a mandatory minimum sentence for black people as for white people charged with the same offense.[6]

These circumstances didn't occur by accident, and they are definitely not coincidental. At a press conference on June 17, 1971, President Nixon identified drug abuse as "public enemy number one in the United States," and launched what has proven to be a diabolical war on drugs. Nixon's aide who jump-started the drug war in 1971, John Ehrlichman, notoriously confessed in 1999 they had deliberately lied for the distinct purpose of creating a false association between drugs and communities of color. The damage done during the 28-year period between 1971 and 1999, and since then, has left a huge, ugly, open wound on the face of the United States.[7]

But many other countries around the world have also outlawed cannabis. One of the reasons cannabis reform has not been seen in this country is because the US is a party to international drug treaties. However, in February of 2019, global health experts at the United Nations (UN) recommended marijuana and its key components should be formally rescheduled under international drug treaties. This proposal followed earlier recommendations from the World Health Organization (WHO) suggesting CBD should not be scheduled at all under international drug conventions. They recommended the addition of a provision that would read: *"Preparations containing predominantly cannabidiol (CBD) and not more than 0.2 percent of delta-9-tetrahydrocannabidiol (THC) are not under international control."*[8] These are among recent indicators the world is recognizing how cannabis has been erroneously classified as a dangerous drug for decades without merit or sound reason.

The tides of change are swelling in the US, as well. Transformations regarding cannabis are beginning to crawl out of the cocoon they've been holed up in for decades. Not only are hemp and hemp-derived products basically legal, but most states have enacted some form of legal medical marijuana use. Additionally, 18 states plus the District of Columbia have legalized adult-use recreational marijuana, and 27 states have decriminalized it. One of the most frequently cited reasons for legalization and decriminalization is that they help ease disparities in arrests for marijuana-related charges. With increasing regularity, people are understanding how other legal substances, like alcohol and certain prescription drugs, are considerably more dangerous and harmful than cannabis.

Long before hemp was criminalized in the United States, it played a significant role in building this country. The Puritans brought it with them when they arrived in colonial America, and British colonies were required to grow hemp, making it critically important to the New World economy; important enough that farmers were allowed to pay their taxes with it. George Washington grew hemp and encouraged all citizens to "sow hemp widely." Thomas Jefferson bred hemp varieties. But the history of hemp in America actually started before European settlers arrived; it was being grown by Native Americans when the Europeans stepped ashore.

WHAT'S IN A SEED?

Another black hole in the CBD universe is the question of whether hemp seed oil and CBD oil are the same thing? The answer to this question surprises many, because it is a resounding NO! Hemp seed oil has no CBD in it.

CBD oil is made by extracting cannabidiol from the flowers, leaves, stems, and stalks of hemp plants. CBD is one of the numerous cannabinoids in cannabis plants, but there are no cannabinoids in the seeds. Hemp seed oil is a product of the seeds, so there are no cannabinoids in hemp seed oil, including CBD. Hemp seed oil has abundant healthy fats, including GLA and omega 3 & 6, so it tends to be used in beauty and skin care products, but skin care products infused with CBD are not nearly as common. If you think you're buying skin care products containing CBD oil, read the label carefully.

Two oils produced from hemp plants that do contain CBD are:

1. **Full-Spectrum CBD Oil**, which contains *all* of the chemical compounds in hemp plants, and

2. **Broad-Spectrum CBD Oil**, which contains all of the chemical compounds in hemp except THC.

FULL-SPECTRUM, BROAD-SPECTRUM, OR ISOLATE?

Full-spectrum CBD oil products contain all the minor cannabinoids, terpenes, lipids, and other molecules from the original hemp plant. People who are subject to drug tests, whether through their employment or for other reasons, need to be aware that full-spectrum hemp-derived CBD products contain a trace amount of THC. Considering hemp products like CBD oil can only have 0.3% THC or less, it is truly a trace amount, but it may be detected in blood and other body fluids. People who are adamant about not taking any THC at all, for any reason, should choose one of the other options.

More and more people are choosing broad-spectrum CBD oil products because they don't have even a trace amount of THC, but only the THC is removed, so broad-spectrum products contain all the minor cannabinoids, terpenes, and other plant material. Broad-spectrum CBD oil products are basically a happy mid-point between full-spectrum products and CBD isolates, since they combine the complete array of phytonutrients from hemp plants except THC.

CBD isolate products contain just one ingredient, CBD. With an isolate product, all the plant remnants, including other cannabinoids, are removed; it is a crystalline solid or powder that is the purest and strongest form of CBD. Though an isolate isn't an oil, the CBD is often suspended in a carrier like hemp seed oil or coconut oil. With an isolate product, there is no risk of triggering a false positive on a drug test. CBD isolate is both tasteless and odorless, and it is easy to measure, so using it is easy and convenient.

3 TYPES OF CBD

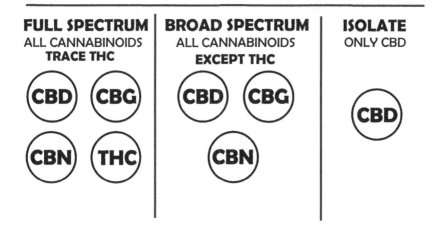

FULL SPECTRUM	BROAD SPECTRUM	ISOLATE
ALL CANNABINOIDS TRACE THC	ALL CANNABINOIDS EXCEPT THC	ONLY CBD
CBD CBG	CBD CBG	CBD
CBN THC	CBN	

WHAT'S IN THE PLANT?

Hemp is a dioecious plant, meaning male and female plants are distinctly different; female hemp plants have seed-producing flowers which form clusters that grow on the pistillate, and male plants have pollen-producing flowers that form on the staminate. Some people incorrectly believe hemp is the male cannabis plant and marijuana is the female, but this is not true. All cannabis species, including hemp, are either female or male (with a few exceptions of hermaphrodites). Female plants are grown to full maturity and harvested at the end of the season; male plants die shortly after pollination.

How to Identify Male and Female Hemp Plants

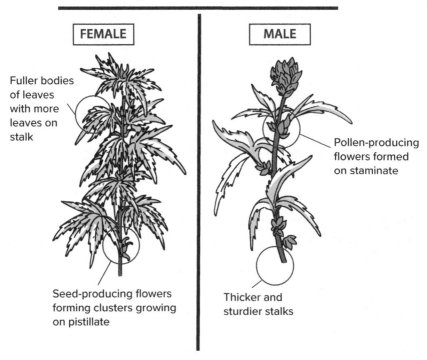

FEMALE

Fuller bodies
of leaves
with more
leaves on
stalk

MALE

Pollen-producing
flowers formed
on staminate

Seed-producing flowers
forming clusters growing
on pistillate

Thicker and
sturdier stalks

Currently, many countries, including the US, differentiate hemp from marijuana by the amount of THC produced *per dry weight of the plant*. This is an interesting and confusing measurement, though, because the content of cannabinoids, including both CBD and THC, varies depending on what part of the plant is used for the dry weight assessment. According to the United Nations Office of Drugs and Crime (UNOD), *"the THC content varies in the different parts of the plant: from 10-12 percent in flowers, 1-2 percent in leaves, 0.1-0.3 percent in stalks, to less than 0.03 percent in the roots."*[9] Clearly, the ratio of different parts of the plant being used for the assessment can make a pretty significant difference. And to further complicate things, there is no official industry standard for calculating the total amount of THC in hemp, so different producers and testing facilities calculate it in different ways.

These are a couple examples of the confusing circumstances that are present throughout the industry.

Despite the challenges of the industry, though, farmers have been enthusiastically growing hemp since it became legal with the passing of the 2018 Farm Bill. Hemp is considered an appealing rotation crop because it detoxifies the soil and prevents erosion while recycling valuable nutrients back into the ground, plus it requires very little water, so it is more environmentally friendly than most traditional crops. Hemp strains are bred for a range of qualities including their resistance to disease, time of harvest, seed production, hemp oil content, and cannabinoid content.

Hemp plants are super-accumulators, meaning they absorb everything in the ground where they are farmed. If the hemp was grown in soil containing even a trace of heavy metals, the resulting oils will contain those heavy metals. This is also true for other toxins like pesticides and herbicides, and chemical fertilizers. Obviously, pollutants like these would contaminate CBD oil products. When buying CBD products, always find out where the hemp was farmed. We recommend choosing hemp raised in the US because hemp and hemp-farmers are very carefully overseen and regulated at both the state and federal levels.

EXTRACTION METHODS

Equally important as knowing where the hemp came from is knowing the effects different extraction methods can have on CBD oil. Both factors are important for determining the quality of the final product. Different extraction methods can have dramatically different outcomes.

Being informed about the methods of CBD extraction is important while the market remains unregulated because, unfortunately, there are some shady companies making false claims about the contents of their products. Like any unregulated industry, the market has become infused with scam artists anxious to make a quick buck, turning the industry into somewhat of a dog-and-pony show by marketing and selling products that are not what they claim to be. Several recent studies have consistently found CBD consumers are not necessarily getting what they thought they were buying. One study by a highly respected research firm found 70% of top-selling CBD products were "highly contaminated."[10] Another report indicated several manufacturers misrepresented the contents of their products. These findings are not isolated, leaving consumers confused and vulnerable.

There are several methods for extracting oil from plants, and different methods can be used for different purposes. A few methods are used to extract CBD, and reputable manufacturers will always provide information about the method they use. Please know these extraction operations are manned by trained professionals using very expensive professional-grade equipment, not by average folks at home in their garage or basement. In other words, don't try this yourself at home!

One method is solvent extraction, where ethanol (highly purified alcohol) is used to separate and extract CBD from the hemp plants. Ethanol is ideal for extracting the full range of plant compounds like terpenes and cannabinoids, but it also extracts chlorophyll. The chlorophyll can be removed through filtering, but the process significantly lowers the potency. Butane is a stronger solvent than ethanol, but it is more likely to have contaminants that taint the final product, potentially causing negative side effects. Additionally, trace amounts of butane solvent remain in the finished product. In order for the finished product to be considered fit for sale, the residue levels must remain under 0.5%. We find it interesting that the acceptable amount of butane solvent is almost twice as high as the legal limit for THC, and we mention this to emphasize how small the trace amount of THC really is in hemp products. You can legally buy products that have a higher content of butane, a known toxin, than the level of THC. Solvent extraction is suitable for high yields of CBD isolates, but not for broad-spectrum or full-spectrum CBD oil because it damages phytochemicals and terpenes.

Another popular extraction method is carbon dioxide (CO_2) extraction, which is the safest and most common method. This process uses pressurized CO_2 to extract phytochemicals from the hemp, and it is sub-divided into three categories: supercritical, mid-critical, and subcritical. CO_2 is a gas at room temperature, but when heated and converted to liquid, it works as a natural solvent and breaks down raw hemp.

Supercritical extractions are more efficient than mid- and subcritical for giving higher yields of CBD, but the higher temperatures damage phytochemicals during the process. Mid-critical and subcritical use lower temperatures, leaving phytochemicals intact, but less of the hemp is actually turned into CBD, so the yield is lower. CO_2 is a non-toxic, natural substance, so any residue is considered safe for human consumption.[11]

CLOSING THOUGHTS

Cannabis, both hemp and marijuana, has seen plenty of tumultuous times in the US over the past several decades. From its protracted sentence as an illegal substance, to the *War on Drugs'* racist beginnings and implementation that are only now being examined and recognized for what they were, modern cultures have worked hard to erase this plant's lengthy history of medicinal promise. Currently, CBD is experiencing a renaissance, including renewed excitement about its therapeutic potential, with impressive results.

As CBD continues growing in popularity, many people remain confused about the differences between cannabis, marijuana, and hemp. Though hemp and marijuana are both cannabis plants, there are many differences between them, including the fact that hemp has no use as a recreational drug. Hemp has just a trace amount of THC, one of at least a hundred chemical compounds, called cannabinoids, found in cannabis plants. THC is the compound that causes the high associated with marijuana use, and because its presence in hemp is so low, hemp-derived CBD products do not cause that high.

Farmers see hemp as an attractive agricultural crop because it recycles nutrients back into the soil and it requires considerably less water than most crops. Growing hemp in organic conditions is critically important because it is a hyper-accumulator, so it absorbs any toxins in the soil. After the hemp is harvested, there are a few different methods used to extract the CBD oil from the plants, and they have different effects on the resulting products.

Knowing which questions to ask at the CBD store can be complicated and confusing. Wherever you are on your personal wellness journey, we believe information is power. You would probably not be reading this book if you were not considering the possibility of including CBD as part of your personal wellness regimen, and you are certainly not alone. Multitudes of people living with multitudes of health issues have benefitted from taking CBD oil. Many of them have been through long periods of time when they were ill and were told nothing more could be done for them. Or even worse, they were left baffled without a diagnosis, and therefore without any kind of treatment protocol. These circumstances, and others like them, are incredibly difficult for people to live with. In response, people are exploring options to help them on their wellness journeys, including CBD oil.

BOLD EXPLORERS
BLAZING THE TRAIL

ROBBIE IS A CANCER SLAYER! And he is definitely Not Done Yet! Diagnosed with Non-Hodgkins lymphoma 20 years ago, Robbie credits Cannabis Medicine, including CBD, with helping him remain cancer free since his initial diagnosis.

His family has been ravaged by cancer. His sister, wife, and one of his three daughters are all breast cancer survivors. His daughter has beaten it twice. Her husband is now fighting esophageal cancer. Robbie's family has lost his brother and his sister's husband to cancer as well. How much cancer can one family endure?

Robbie has been a consumer of cannabis products for their medicinal value since the days when they were not legal in any form or capacity. The first time his daughter was fighting breast cancer was prior to 2018, so not even hemp-derived CBD was available legally, and medical marijuana was not available in their state. It broke his heart to see her losing her beautiful hair and vomiting up the medication that was supposed to kill her cancer. Wanting desperately to help ease some of her pain, he suggested she try cannabis for the nausea. She refused out of fear that if the police found out she was using cannabis, she would be at risk of having her children taken away.

What a despicable choice — ease the horrible side effects of your cancer medication, or keep your children. Unfortunately, that choice has been reality for millions of people.

Robbie has dedicated every breath he takes to eradicating cancer, or at least some of the pain involved with treating it. He's been a volunteer in the cancer ward at his local hospital for years. He shares the stories of others who have beaten this awful disease, believing it offers the patients inspiration and a reason to keep up their own fight. He runs a Facebook page for cancer patients, and he hosts a podcast for cancer patients called "Not Done Yet." He believes in early detection and treatment, and he feels that getting positive messages into the world is a good way to help people through their fear of being diagnosed with cancer.

At one point, Robbie decided to come clean about using cannabis. Luckily, when he told the hospital where he volunteers and offered to quit if they thought he should, they did not ask him to resign. They simply asked him not to offer it to the patients. So, he continues bringing love and light onto the cancer ward. Since then, Robbie has convinced his cancer hospital that it is in the best interest of their Illinois patients to have legal access to medical cannabis. "I simply told them over and over 'if your patients can eat better and sleep better, they're going to fight better!'" They eventually believed him.

When you talk with Robbie, you immediately get a sense of sheer positivity. He describes himself as both grateful and content, and he is a big believer in creating change by using positive words. He knows first-hand how receiving a cancer diagnosis causes people to lose their sense of purpose and their identity. He works at offering them a sense of purpose and value. Robbie is quick to acknowledge the people who inspire him, and he has a personal goal to climb Mount Kilimanjaro.

Robbie lives with chemo-induced neuropathy to the extent that he hasn't been able to make a fist for a very long time. After taking the CBD tincture for just a couple of days, he could close his hand better than he's been able to since he had the cancer and the chemo. He uses CBD balm on his knees, calves, hands, and shoulders, and describes not only that it has helped ease his chronic pain, but has offered him increased mobility and range of motion.

Knowing what a positive effect he gets from the CBD, he suggested it to a friend who lives with anxiety and insomnia. She is thrilled with how much better it makes her feel.

He also suggested the CBD balm to a friend living with such a painful bunion that he could barely walk. This friend got so much pain relief he was able to get up on his roof and do some repairs that had been needed, but he couldn't be on his feet long enough to get it done.

Robbie's son is a teacher and a coach, so Robbie helped him get a broad-spectrum product without any THC, and now he has far fewer aches and pains.

Robbie, you are definitely Not Done Yet! Keep up the good work, keep fighting on behalf of those who are facing their own cancer battles, continue slaying the cancer!

Chapter

2

THE FARM BILL was signed into law on December 20, 2018, effectively removing hemp from Schedule 1 of the Controlled Substances Act (CSA), as long as it is farmed by licensed growers in accordance with all the terms of the new law. Hemp had been illegal since the implementation of the Marihuana Tax Act in 1937, and it was placed on Schedule 1 of the CSA in 1970. In response, advocates who believe in Cannabis Medicine have been working since 1971 to have cannabis removed from Schedule 1, a category for drugs, substances, or chemicals with no currently accepted medical use and a high potential for abuse. Many people, especially Cannabis Medicine advocates, were excited when the Farm Bill was signed and became law.

At the time, there was some concern among people working in the industry, though, that the FDA might take the initiative to develop regulations that would impose significant, strict limitations. So far, the FDA has declined to establish any guidelines at all for CBD products, and the absence of federal oversight has left the market somewhat of a free-for-all. So, like bold, visionary trail blazers always do, industry leaders have been working diligently to develop policies and strategies for managing the market within the framework of the Farm Bill in order for it to grow and prosper.

People in the hemp/CBD industry have worked tirelessly to earn the public's trust. One strategy they've implemented has legitimate CBD companies offering layers of security to their customers through web-based platforms providing access to important information about their products. Additionally, the industry has established standards for labeling products, and offers guidance on how to read and interpret the labels so that consumers can understand what they're buying – and what they're not buying (like THC), as the case might be.

WHAT'S IN THE BOTTLE?

Particularly in the absence of federal guidelines, CBD consumers need to be discerning readers of CBD product labels, which vary from one state to another. While certain CBD labels may be compliant with the requirements of multiple states, there are no CBD product labels in full compliance with the requirements in all states. However, when two states first developed and implemented legal adult-use, recreational marijuana programs, the federal government developed recommendations for the legal marijuana industry, and those recommendations are now being viewed as trail markers for navigating the hemp/CBD industry.

Marijuana remains illegal at the federal level, but in 2013, Colorado and Washington became the first states to begin operating legal, regulated, adult-use recreational marijuana programs. These voter-approved programs forced state and federal governments to work together in new ways, and one of the strategies states have adopted to successfully navigate the hemp/CBD industry is by following the recommendations of a federal document known as the *Cole Memo*.

In August 2013, then-Attorney General James M. Cole issued a memorandum to all US Attorney Generals. Now known as the *Cole Memo*, this document, published by the Department of Justice, established guidelines for the federal government, state governments, and law enforcement to work together within legal adult-use recreational marijuana programs. These are the guidelines being used as guideposts by leaders in the CBD industry.[12]

Basically, the *Cole Memo* told states if they implemented strict regulatory frameworks and seed-to-sale tracking systems to monitor the growth, distribution, and sales of regulated cannabis, and created a transparent, accountable market, the federal government would leave them alone. The Obama-era Cole Memo was revoked by President Trump's Department of Justice in January 2018, but at least one high-level authority from the Trump administration was quoted as stating, *"there is validity to the Cole Memo,"* which was widely interpreted to mean the safest way to participate in the industry was to remain compliant with its recommendations. Industry leaders believe the Biden-administration's Department of Justice will reinstate the Cole Memo, and will likely craft new additional guidance defining enforcement standards.

Compliant cannabis companies, including those manufacturing CBD products, have designed software packages to implement traceability systems for seed-to-sale by licensed commercial cannabis businesses and government regulatory bodies. These software packages provide transparent inventory management and seed-to-sale tracking data, bringing layers of accountability to all the activities of licensed businesses.

Every state also requires, in one way or another, the labels of CBD products meet the requirements of the federal Food, Drug and Cosmetic Act (FDCA). Under the FDCA, the labels for product sold in the US must contain four basic elements:

- An identity statement indicating what the product is,
- A net weight statement,
- A list of all ingredients,
- The name and address of the manufacturer, packer, or distributor.[13]

Furthermore, a growing number of states are requiring QR code links, scannable bar codes, or web addresses linked to documents that provide the following information:

- The batch identification number,
- The product name,
- The batch date,
- The expiration date, which in some states must be no more than two years from the date of manufacture,
- The batch size,
- The total quantity produced,
- The ingredients,
- A certificate of analysis.

Several states require labels for CBD products to include the following statement: *"The FDA has not evaluated this product for safety or efficacy."*[14]

THIRD PARTY EVALUATION

For consumers, deciding which CBD products to purchase can be challenging, even for those who have done their homework thoroughly. To that end, one of the steps being used to manage the market in the absence of federal oversight is third party evaluation, or having an independent, unbiased analysis and report of the contents of a company's CBD products. This is incredibly important in today's market, because the lack of federal oversight has essentially left the door wide open for some businesses to engage in sales tactics that are not particularly impressive with regard to ethical business practices.

Third-party testing has become critically important in today's market because it provides unbiased analyses of quality, purity, and potency from samples of legitimate CBD products being sold. Until the FDA develops guidelines for CBD products, the door remains wide open for manufacturers to misrepresent the contents of their products, and this is where third-party testing comes in. CBD manufacturers send samples of each of their products to a laboratory that independently analyzes them and then reports the results. Manufacturers post these lab results for each batch online to confirm that the information listed on product labels accurately represents the contents of the product.

Many labs have earned good reputations within the industry for providing consistent, accurate test results. The most common tests run by third-party labs are cannabinoid profiles. Using specialized testing techniques, the concentration of cannabinoids can be used to confirm the amount of CBD listed on the bottle is accurate. Cannabinoid profiles are also important to establish the presence or absence of THC, and the ratio of terpenes and other elements are also reported. Third-party labs also test for heavy metals and for biological contaminants like herbicides and pesticides, and chemical fertilizers.

CERTIFICATE OF ANALYSIS (COA)

A Certificate of Analysis (COA) is a document from an accredited laboratory confirming the contents of the product. Once you've tentatively decided on the product you want to purchase, there should be a QR code on the label that, when scanned, will link you directly to a webpage with the product's COA. Reputable manufacturers send a sample from every batch of every product they make to a lab for testing in order to verify the labels accurately represent the contents of the products. Although QR codes are not required on CBD product labels in all states, they are the accepted standard for the industry. All reputable companies want their CBD product information readily available to their customers. If you can't access a COA from a product label, that's definitely not a good sign. Keep shopping and choose a different product.

There are several important elements to reading and interpreting a COA. Here are five steps to help you make sense of what can seem like a complicated document:

1. Check the name of the laboratory that ran the tests.
   Verify the laboratory that ran the test results is an independent operation. Confirm the laboratory is accredited and abides by industry standards and best practices.

2. Ensure the batch number on the COA and on the product match.
   The batch number refers to the CBD products that were made with a specific "batch" of CBD extract. The COA batch number must match the batch number on your CBD product label to be relevant.

3. Read the cannabinoid profile.
   Compare the cannabinoid content listed in the test results to the profile listed on the product label; they should match or be very close to what is on the label.

4. Pay attention to the heavy metals analysis.
   Always check the COA to confirm heavy metal testing was performed and that the CBD product is either free of these substances or within defined safety limits.

5. Examine the herbicide/pesticide analysis list.
   Review the COA to ensure they've tested for pesticides and herbicides.

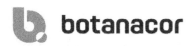**botanacor**

prepared for: GLACIERPAK LLC
1070 DIAMOND VALLEY DRIVE, SUITE 200
WINDSOR, CO 80550

Tincture: 30 mL, 1800 mg

Batch ID:	BR-112-T30-18-211207-00	**Test ID:**	T000189392
Type:	Unit	**Submitted:**	01/25/2022 @ 01:46 PM
Test:	Potency	**Started:**	1/26/2022
Method:	TM14 (HPLC-DAD)	**Reported:**	1/28/2022

CANNABINOID PROFILE

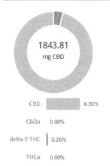

1843.81 mg CBD

CBD 6.30%

CBDa 0.00%

delta 9 THC 0.26%

THCa 0.00%

Compound	LOQ (mg)	Result (mg)	Result (mg/g)
Delta 9-Tetrahydrocannabinolic acid (THCA-A)	3.39	ND	ND
Delta 9-Tetrahydrocannabinol (Delta 9THC)	3.83	76.42	2.6
Cannabidiolic acid (CBDA)	4.30	ND	ND
Cannabidiol (CBD)	4.19	1843.81	63.0
Delta 8-Tetrahydrocannabinol (Delta 8THC)	4.22	ND	ND
Cannabinolic Acid (CBNA)	2.42	ND	ND
Cannabinol (CBN)	1.10	94.53	3.2
Cannabigerolic acid (CBGA)	3.54	ND	ND
Cannabigerol (CBG)	0.85	73.31	2.5
Tetrahydrocannabivarinic Acid (THCVA)	2.99	ND	ND
Tetrahydrocannabivarin (THCV)	0.77	ND	ND
Cannabidivarinic Acid (CBDVA)	1.79	ND	ND
Cannabidivarin (CBDV)	0.99	11.33	0.4
Cannabichromenic Acid (CBCA)	1.36	ND	ND
Cannabichromene (CBC)	1.49	91.39	3.1
Total Cannabinoids		**2190.79**	**74.9**
Total Potential THC**		76.42	2.6
Total Potential CBD**		1843.81	63.0

% = % (w/w) = Percent Weight of Analyte / Weight of Product
* Total Cannabinoids result reflects the absolute sum of all
cannabinoids detected
** Total Potential THC/CBD is calculated using the following formulas
to take into account the loss of a carboxyl group during
decarboxylation step:
Total THC = THC + (THCa *(0.877)) and
Total CBD = CBD + (CBDa *(0.877))
ND = None Detected (Defined by Dynamic Range of the method)

NOTES:
# of Servings = 1, Sample Weight=29.25g

FINAL APPROVAL

Daniel Weidensaul		Daniel Weidensaul 28-Jan-2022 2:08 PM
	K Winternheimer	Karen Winternheime 28-Jan-2022 2:16 PM
PREPARED BY / DATE	APPROVED BY / DATE	

Certificate #4329.02

Botanacor Laboratories™, All Rights Reserved | 1301 S Jason St Unit K, Denver, CO 80223 | 888.800.8223 | www.botanacor.com

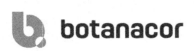

botanacor

CERTIFICATE OF ANALYSIS

prepared for: GLACIERPAK LLC
1070 DIAMOND VALLEY DRIVE, SUITE 200
WINDSOR, CO 80550

BR-112-T30-10-200924-15

Batch ID:	FS 1000 30 mL	**Test ID:**	T000103854
Type:	Unit	**Submitted:**	10/16/2020 @ 04:34 PM
Test:	Potency	**Started:**	10/20/2020
Method:	TM14	**Reported:**	10/21/2020

CANNABINOID PROFILE

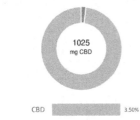

1025 mg CBD

CBD ███████ 3.50%

CBDa 0.01%

delta 9 THC | 0.07%

THCa 0.00%

Compound	LOQ (mg)	Result (mg)	Result (mg/g)
Delta 9-Tetrahydrocannabinolic acid (THCA-A)	6.28	ND	ND
Delta 9-Tetrahydrocannabinol (Delta 9THC)	3.08	20.05	0.7
Cannabidiolic acid (CBDA)	1.77	3.23	0.1
Cannabidiol (CBD)	3.77	1025.00	35.0
Delta 8-Tetrahydrocannabinol (Delta 8THC)	3.36	ND	ND
Cannabinolic Acid (CBNA)	8.71	ND	ND
Cannabinol (CBN)	3.82	33.45	1.1
Cannabigerolic acid (CBGA)	5.49	ND	ND
Cannabigerol (CBG)	3.07	53.21	1.8
Tetrahydrocannabivarinic Acid (THCVA)	5.35	ND	ND
Tetrahydrocannabivarin (THCV)	2.74	ND	ND
Cannabidivarinic Acid (CBDVA)	1.70	ND	ND
Cannabidivarin (CBDV)	0.91	3.83	0.1
Cannabichromenic Acid (CBCA)	4.82	ND	ND
Cannabichromene (CBC)	5.57	44.48	1.5
Total Cannabinoids		1183.25	40.5
Total Potential THC**		20.05	0.7
Total Potential CBD**		1027.83	35.1

NOTES:

# of Servings = 1, Sample Weight=29.25g

N/A

% = % (w/w) – Percent (Weight of Analyte - Weight of Product)
* Total Cannabinoids result reflects the absolute sum of all cannabinoids detected.
** Total Potential THC/CBD is calculated using the following formulas
   to take into account the loss of a carboxyl group during
   decarboxylation step.
   Total THC = THC + (THCa *0.877) and
   Total CBD = CBD + (CBDa *0.877)
ND = None Detected (Defined by Dynamic Range of the method)

FINAL APPROVAL

	Daniel Weidensaul 21-Oct-2020 4:58 PM		Greg Zimpfer 21-Oct-2020 5:34 PM
PREPARED BY / DATE		**APPROVED BY / DATE**	

Certificate #4329.02

Botanacor Laboratories™, All Rights Reserved | 1301 S Jason St Unit K, Denver, CO 80223 | 888.800.8223 | www.botanacor.com

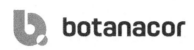 **botanacor**

CERTIFICATE OF ANALYSIS

prepared for: GLACIERPAK LLC
1070 DIAMOND VALLEY DRIVE, SUITE 200
WINDSOR, CO 80550

BR-112-T30-06-200924-14

Batch ID:	FS 600 30 mL	Test ID:	T000103853
Type:	Unit	Submitted:	10/16/2020 @ 04:34 PM
Test:	Potency	Started:	10/20/2020
Method:	TM14	Reported:	10/21/2020

CANNABINOID PROFILE

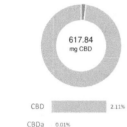

617.84
mg CBD

CBD		2.11%
CBDa	0.01%	
delta 9 THC	0.04%	
THCa	0.00%	

% = % (w/a) - Percent (Weight of Analyte : Weight of Product)
* Total Cannabinoids result reflects the absolute sum of all cannabinoids detected
** Total Potential THC/CBD is calculated using the following formulas
to take into account the loss of a carboxy group during
decarboxylation step.
Total THC = THC + (THCa *(0.877)) and
Total CBD = CBD + (CBDa *(0.877))
ND = None Detected (Defined by Dynamic Range of the method)

Compound	LOQ (mg)	Result (mg)	Result (mg/g)
Delta 9-Tetrahydrocannabinolic acid (THCA-A)	6.28	ND	ND
Delta 9-Tetrahydrocannabinol (Delta 9THC)	3.08	10.84	0.4
Cannabidiolic acid (CBDA)	1.77	2.16	0.1
Cannabidiol (CBD)	3.77	617.84	21.1
Delta 8-Tetrahydrocannabinol (Delta 8THC)	3.36	ND	ND
Cannabinolic Acid (CBNA)	8.71	ND	ND
Cannabinol (CBN)	3.82	23.18	0.8
Cannabigerolic acid (CBGA)	5.48	ND	ND
Cannabigerol (CBG)	3.07	32.07	1.1
Tetrahydrocannabivarinic Acid (THCVA)	5.35	ND	ND
Tetrahydrocannabivarin (THCV)	2.74	ND	ND
Cannabidivarinic Acid (CBDVA)	1.70	ND	ND
Cannabidivarin (CBDV)	0.91	2.00	0.1
Cannabichromenic Acid (CBCA)	4.82	ND	ND
Cannabichromene (CBC)	5.57	27.50	0.9
Total Cannabinoids		**715.59**	**24.5**
Total Potential THC**		10.84	0.4
Total Potential CBD**		619.73	21.2

NOTES:
# of Servings = 1, Sample Weight=29.25g

N/A

FINAL APPROVAL

Daniel Weidensaul
21-Oct-2020
4:58 PM

PREPARED BY / DATE

Greg Zimpfer
21-Oct-2020
5:34 PM

APPROVED BY / DATE

ilac-MRA
ACCREDITED
Certificate #4329.02

Botanacor Laboratories™, All Rights Reserved | 1301 S Jason St Unit K, Denver, CO 80223 | 888.800.8223 | www.botanacor.com

READING PRODUCT LABELS

Whether you're shopping online or down the street at your neighborhood CBD store, knowing how to read and understand the product labels will help guide you through the labyrinth of CBD products and hopefully choose one that will best meet your goals. There are some standard listings on legitimate CBD product labels. For example, all labels for reputable products include the following:

- The name of the manufacturer and/or the distributor,
- Information about the suggested serving size, the number of servings per unit, and the number of servings per package,
- How much hemp oil is in each serving,
- How much CBD is in each serving, and if the product also contains THC, the amount per serving will also be provided,
- The type of CBD Oil,

    Hemp-derived CBD products are made with either full-spectrum CBD oil, broad-spectrum CBD oil, or CBD isolate. All three are natural and originate with hemp, but they can contain a variety of other compounds.

- Other Ingredients,

    CBD oil can be infused into or mixed with other compounds to create products like tinctures and edibles. The labels for these products will contain a list of all other ingredients.

- Expiration Date.

    *CBD oil products tend to be long-lasting, but CBD does degrade over time (natural CBD products will last longer because flavorings degrade faster than the actual CBD).

Because there are no federal guidelines for CBD product labels, there is a pretty wide range of labeling requirements from state to state. And just to make things even more complicated, within any given state, different labels from different brands and products don't necessarily look the same. Even people who've been immersed in the CBD industry for a long time can find it difficult and overwhelming when trying to compare products.

MOVING FORWARD

The times are definitely changing in positive ways for people in the cannabis industry. By late summer of 2019, dozens of cannabis policy reform bills had been introduced in state legislatures across the country, and several seemed poised to pass. Then the COVID-19 pandemic reared its ugly head and states halted their legislative sessions, placing most of these bills on the back burner. Now that state legislatures are back in business, it will be interesting to see how these bills proceed through the systems. In the meantime, 2021 proved to be an exciting time for the cannabis industry:

- The Drug War is America's longest and perhaps most deadly war. Just ahead of the June 17, 2021 50th anniversary of Nixon's declaration of the War on Drugs, members of the House of Representatives unveiled the Drug Policy Reform Act (DPRA). In addition to eliminating criminal penalties at the federal level for drug possession, the bill provides incentives for state and local governments to adopt decriminalization policies or have their eligibility for funds in grant programs limited. The proposal ends the threat of incarceration for people facing charges of possessing drugs for personal use. Importantly, the DPRA will create a "Commission on Substance Use, Health, and Safety" under the Department of Health and Human Services (HHS) to determine benchmarks using evidence-based solutions. Finally, under the DPRA, individuals impacted by the War on Drugs will be able to seal past records, restore voting rights, and regain access to federal benefits like SNAP nutrition assistance, TANF, and housing assistance. The measure proposes making HHS, rather than the Justice Department, responsible for classifying drugs, shifting that role to a health-centric model.[15],[16]

- In May of 2021, the DEA announced it had reached an important point in the process of increasing the amount of cannabis available for scientific research. They issued a memorandum of agreement to multiple growers, essentially stating these growers are in compliance with federal laws and regulations concerning producing cannabis for research. This is significant, because there has been only one grower licensed with the federal government to produce cannabis for legal scientific research.[17]

- Also in May of 2021, a pair of congressional Republican lawmakers introduced a bill to federally legalize marijuana, protect banks that service state-legal cannabis businesses, and ensure military veterans are specifically permitted to use marijuana in compliance with state laws. The main crux of the legislation is to federally de-schedule cannabis with language on legal protections and mandates for federal studies using medical cannabis. However, it does not contain social justice provisions to repair the past harms of the War on Drugs.[18]

Several states have enacted their own regulatory standards regarding the sale of CBD products under state law. For example, while California's Department of Public Health has adopted the FDA's position that CBD is not permitted in food and beverages, other states have issued their own regulatory policies regarding the sale of hemp-derived products. Regulations continue to evolve in each state as state legislators work to determine a balance between competing interests. Businesses expect local cannabis regulations to continue evolving as the industry grows and recognize they must be able to adapt to this unpredictable regulatory landscape.

APPROVED – OR NOT?

One black hole that has caused a lot of confusion around CBD products is the question of whether they are FDA-approved? So far, only one CBD-based medication, Epidiolex, has been approved by the FDA. Epidiolex is a treatment for seizures associated with rare forms of pediatric epilepsy, and it is the very first medication the FDA has ever approved containing a natural compound from cannabis plants. Many people are excited and hopeful about the possibility of CBD being used for other pharmaceutical medications in the future, now the first one has made its way through the approval process.

Epidiolex was approved in June, 2018, then a short time later, researchers from the University of Arkansas Medical Sciences found high doses of CBD caused liver damage in mice.[19] Critics of the study argued the dosage used in this study was so extremely high it was equal to "the allometrically scaled mouse equivalent of the maximum recommended human maintenance dose." The FDA published a consumer update a year later, in June, 2019, stating they didn't yet know enough about the safety of CBD and warned that liver damage could be one of the side effects from taking CBD.[20] The report provides no explanation of how or why they reached these conclusions.

Interestingly, during clinical trials for Epidiolex, researchers found the medication caused liver toxicity in a few of the patients, who were promptly removed from the study. The endorsement process continued, and ultimately ended in approval, so today Epidiolex is a valid treatment option for children suffering from specific types of epilepsy. There are children in the US being administered regular, ongoing CBD treatments comparable to the amounts given to mice in the Arkansas study, with the full blessing of the FDA.

Though Epidiolex is the first approved naturally occurring cannabinoid therapy, there are two other medications, Marinol and Syndros, made with the active ingredient dronabinol,[21] a synthetic version of THC, and both are FDA approved for certain specific uses. Another FDA-approved drug, Cesamet, contains the active ingredient nabilone,[22] another synthetic chemical remarkably similar to THC. Clearly, the FDA recognizes there is medicinal promise with both CBD and THC, though further approvals remain to be seen. In the meantime, the FDA is holding firm on their position that

CBD is not a pharmaceutical drug because it is not used to diagnose, cure, treat, or prevent disease.[23]

This is just one example of many ironies between the US federal government and the cannabis industry. As mentioned in the introduction, we are not interested in painting a negative picture of the government and/or any of its agencies or departments, but we do want to clear the muck of confusing information about CBD. For the FDA to approve CBD as a treatment for epilepsy, then turn around and deny recognizing it as a "treatment" leaves us scratching our heads and asking, "Huh?"

But where can we turn for accurate information about CBD if not the FDA? Some have suggested the Department of Health and Human Services (HHS), the federal government's agency that works, *"To enhance the health and well-being of all Americans, by providing for effective health and human services and by fostering sound, sustained advances in the sciences underlying medicine, public health, and social services."*[24] Although this might seem like a good place to start, upon further examination, we're skeptical.

Removing cannabis from Schedule 1 has been proposed repeatedly since 1971. At a congressional hearing in June, 2014, the Deputy Director for Regulatory Programs at the FDA said the agency was conducting an analysis, at the request of the DEA, on whether cannabis should be downgraded. Then, in August, 2016, the DEA re-established its long-standing position and again denied removing cannabis from Schedule 1. And thus, the perpetual cycle of proposals to remove cannabis from Schedule 1 continues.

However, the US Patent Office issued patent #6630507 to HHS on October 10, 2003 listing the use of specific cannabinoids, including CBD, as useful in treating neurodegenerative conditions and diseases. A summary included with the application, the abstract for this patent, reads:

"Cannabinoids have been found to have antioxidant properties, unrelated to NMDA receptor antagonism. This new found property

makes cannabinoids useful in the treatment and prophylaxis of a wide variety of oxidation associated diseases, such as ischemic, age-related, inflammatory and autoimmune diseases. The cannabinoids are found to have particular application as neuroprotectants, for example in limiting neurological damage following ischemic insults, such as stroke and trauma, or in the treatment of neurodegenerative diseases, such as Alzheimer's disease, Parkinson's disease and HIV dementia. Nonpsychoactive cannabinoids, such as cannabidiol, are particularly advantageous to use because they avoid toxicity encountered with psychoactive cannabinoids at high doses useful in the method of the present invention."[25]

The patent is limited to certain non-psychoactive compounds in cannabis, and CBD is mentioned several times. The patent also states: *"No signs of toxicity or serious side effects have been observed following chronic administration of cannabidiol to healthy volunteers, even in large acute doses."*[26]

There is absolutely no way to interpret this information other than the government does, in fact, know certain compounds in cannabis, including CBD, have medicinal qualities and they are not harmful for human consumption. There goes any argument for leaving cannabis under Schedule 1!

The research arm of HHS is the National Institutes of Health (NIH), which conducts research about health-related innovations and new discoveries. The NIH states they apply for patents related to their research in order to generate products and services that will benefit public health. These patents allow scientists at the NIH to control the research while directing other entities to actually conduct the tests. Scientists with the NIH were researching antioxidant qualities to help ease degenerative brain diseases when they applied for the patent on cannabinoids. The main reason for the patent is to allow the NIH to contract with an outside company to continue the research – but only according to stipulations set by the NIH.

A New York-based company, Kannalife Sciences Inc., was the only licensee of patent #6630507, with an exclusive license from the NIH to use the technology outlined in the patent to develop cannabinoid-based medications. The agreement also states HHS will receive a percentage of royalties when Kannalife Sciences starts making money from the products developed through this research. All of sudden, HHS doesn't really look like an unbiased source of information about CBD.

These are a few of the reasons we wanted to write this book. Consumers, and those who are simply curious about CBD, have a very difficult time sorting through the vast amount of information, much of which is less than straight forward, as these examples show. Between the partial information, mis-information, mixed messages, and propaganda being spewed by scammers interested in making a quick buck, it is easy to see why people are confused. Consider that many people know CBD was "legalized" in 2018 by the Farm Bill, but very few even know what the Farm Bill is, let alone what it actually says. Rumors are rampant, fanning the flames of misinformation, but legitimate information is awfully difficult to find, analyze, interpret, and use.

CLARIFICATION, PLEASE

In an effort to bring clarification to some of the confusion created by the 2018 Farm Bill, the US Department of Agriculture (USDA) established "interim final rules" for the production of hemp, which were published in the Federal Register on October 31, 2019.[27] Unfortunately, though, the interim rules left plenty of room for clarification. For example, with regard to pre-harvest testing, the rules state: "*Within 15 days prior to the anticipated harvest date, a designated person (from a governmental or law enforcement agency) must collect samples of the crop.*"[28] While this requirement appears simple enough on the surface, it could end up having important ramifications if the state agency doing the sampling fails to collect the sample in the allotted time frame. The USDA itself states that collecting a sample later than planned could produce test results with higher THC content, because all cannabis plants, including hemp, convert other cannabinoids into THC as they approach maturity and harvest. So, realistically, a day or two difference (or more?) in collecting the sample could mean the difference between an entire crop having to be destroyed or not. Timing is critical and the stakes are extremely high.

Additionally, the interim rules allow for some interesting tolerances on the 0.3% THC limit. The rules explicitly state hemp products could test higher than the limit but still qualify as hemp: *"The method used for sampling from the material of the cannabis plant must be sufficient at a confidence level of 95 percent (95%) that no more than one percent (1%) of the plants in the lot would exceed the acceptable hemp THC level."* The Farm Bill goes on to define "acceptable hemp THC level" as: *"When the application of the measurement of uncertainty to the reported delta-9 tetrahydrocannabinol content concentration level on a dry weight basis produces a distribution or range that includes 0.3% or less."*[29]

What?!?!?

We've already established there is no standard method or technique for calculating the THC content in hemp. As loose as this fact is, it becomes further complicated by the fact that when hemp is tested, there is a margin of error in the precision of the result. The margin of error, or "confidence level," must be reported along with the actual result. This creates an interesting and potentially ethical dilemma for the testing laboratories, as they could be "motivated" to keep the results as imprecise as possible. Furthermore, *"Total THC"* is meant to refer to the amount of THC that will be present as a percentage of dry weight after THC-A, another cannabinoid that is a precursor to THC, has been converted into THC. The rules state the testing method must include a validated testing methodology that uses post-decarboxylation, which is defined in the rules as, *"the removal or elimination of a carboxyl group from a molecule or organic compound."*[30]

The cannabinoid THC-A will naturally decarboxylate into THC over time, or immediately after being exposed to heat. So, what this really means is the sample must be heated to convert the non-intoxicating cannabinoid THC-A into THC, but it's awfully difficult to get that message out of the confusing verbiage. These basic examples, drawn directly from the USDA's own interim rules, certainly highlight the point that when it comes to the US government and cannabis, nothing is simple or straight-forward.

Among other things, the 2018 Agriculture Improvement Act (the Farm Bill) changed certain federal rules related to the production and marketing of hemp, and it removed hemp from the Controlled Substances Act, provided it is grown by a licensed grower in accordance with all the requirements of the law. The 2018 Farm Bill allows hemp to be cultivated broadly, and it specifically allows hemp-derived products to be transported across state lines.

The 2018 Farm Bill contains a preemptive provision requiring states to allow interstate transportation of legally produced hemp products, but a few states have argued that transporting hemp, or certain types of hemp-derived products, across their state lines is still illegal. These states don't recognize a distinction between marijuana products and hemp-derived CBD because of the trace amounts of THC in full-spectrum CBD products. So, a hemp-derived CBD product with less than 0.3% THC, as required for it to be considered hemp at the federal level, could still be considered marijuana in certain states. As of 2021 the list of states with such restrictions included Idaho, Kansas, Nebraska, and South Dakota.

There are no federal restrictions on the sale, transport, or possession of hemp-derived products as long as they are produced in a manner consistent with the law. However, the Farm Bill did not create a completely free system where people or businesses can grow however much hemp whenever and wherever they want -- numerous restrictions remain in place.

First of all, hemp cannot contain more than 0.3% THC or it is considered marijuana, and therefore is not eligible for the protections of the Farm

Bill. Second, regulating hemp is now a shared responsibility between each state and the federal government. The Farm Bill required state Departments of Agriculture to work with their respective state's governor and chief law enforcement officer to create a state-specific plan for licensing and regulating hemp, and then submit that plan to the Secretary of the USDA. Any state's plan to license and regulate hemp only became official after it received approval from the Secretary of the USDA. In states that chose not to design a hemp regulatory program, the USDA developed and implemented one that allows hemp farmers in those states to apply for licenses and participate in federally-run programs. Third, the law outlines violations of federal hemp law, including cultivating without a license or producing cannabis with more than 0.3% THC. The law outlines possible punishments for these violations, plus courses of action for violators to become compliant, and defines which activities are considered felonies.[31]

Ultimately, the Farm Bill went a considerable distance in the direction of legalizing hemp, but it did not create a system allowing people to grow it as freely as we can grow corn and soybeans; it is a myth the Farm Bill legalized CBD. The bill adamantly states, *"any product derived from hemp will be legal if, and only if, the hemp is produced by a licensed grower in a manner consistent with the Farm Bill and all associated federal and state regulations."*[32] Hemp remains highly regulated in the United States.

Another black hole has been the question of whether scientists and medical researchers must continue using research-grade hemp from the only federally approved source, the Marijuana Program at the University of Mississippi School of Pharmacy's National Center for Natural Products Research. Because of hemp's long-standing status as a Schedule 1 Controlled Substance, this has been the case for decades.

But on June 30, 2020, the US House of Representatives approved legislation allowing researchers to study cannabis purchased from businesses in state-legal marijuana markets, taking another small step in the direction of federal legalization. Then in May of 2021, the DEA announced it had reached an important point in the process of increasing the amount of cannabis available for scientific research. They issued a memorandum of agreement to multiple growers, essentially stating those growers are in compliance with federal laws and regulations concerning the production of cannabis for research.

THE FDA, FFDCA, AND DSHEA

The FDA regulates both finished dietary supplements and dietary ingredients under a different set of regulations than the ones covering conventional food and drug products. These regulations, known as the Dietary Supplement Health and Education Act of 1994 (DSHEA), provide the FDA with appropriate regulatory authority and enforcement tools to protect consumers while still allowing them access to a wide variety of affordable, high quality, safe, and beneficial dietary supplement products. The DSHEA amends the Federal Food, Drug, and Cosmetic Act of 1938 (FFDCA) to include the way dietary supplements are regulated and labeled.

DSHEA defines the term "dietary supplement" as:

"... any product (other than tobacco) intended to supplement the diet that bears or contains one or more dietary ingredient, including a vitamin, a mineral, an herb or other botanical, an amino acid, a dietary substance for use by man to supplement the diet by increasing the total dietary intake, or a concentrate, metabolite, constituent, extract, or combination of any of the aforementioned ingredients."[33]

Furthermore, a dietary supplement must be labeled as a dietary supplement, be intended for ingestion, and must not be represented for use as conventional food or as the sole item of a meal or of the diet.

Under the act, supplement manufacturers do not need FDA approval to market dietary supplements if they were being marketed in the United States before 1994. However, products that do not qualify to be grandfathered in are defined as *"New Dietary Ingredients,"* and their makers are required to provide reasonable evidence of, or reasonable expectation of, their safety. New Dietary Ingredients must be reviewed (not approved) by the FDA before they can be marketed.

The 2018 Farm Bill had no effect on the FDA's authority to regulate CBD or other hemp products; it also did not change the regulatory definitions of "food additive" and "dietary ingredient" for ingredients like CBD in food and dietary supplements. The FDA has authority to regulate products containing cannabis and cannabis-derived compounds, including those classified as hemp. Therefore, CBD is subject to the same regulatory requirements under the FFDCA as other food additives and new dietary ingredients. The FDA has consistently taken the position that it is unlawful to sell a food or dietary supplement containing CBD because CBD is not eligible for use in those products under the FFDCA because CBD has been studied for "drug" uses, including clinical studies that led to the FDA's 2018 approval of Epidiolex.

The FDA's jurisdiction is triggered by a product's intended use. Generally, the FDA determines intended use based on claims made by a product's manufacturer, which are often included on the product's labeling, or in promotional and advertising materials. If a company states that its product can be used to diagnose, cure, mitigate, treat, or prevent a disease, or that it affects the bodily structure or function of the consumer, the FDA is likely to decide the product is a drug under the FFDCA.

Although research has demonstrated tremendous potential for CBD to help people in remarkable ways, legitimate CBD companies do not make direct medical claims. For a manufacturer of CBD products to make medical claims about their products with regard to treating any medical condition or symptom is a strict violation of the FFDCA/DSHEA guidelines.[34]

CLOSING THOUGHTS

These are interesting and exciting times for people working in the hemp/CBD industry. 2021 continued bringing changes that left Cannabis Medicine advocates optimistic. In the meantime, the FDA, for the first time ever, has approved a cannabinoid-based medication. Epidiolex is officially approved as a treatment for specific forms of pediatric epilepsy. With this approval, many people are hopeful for approvals of additional cannabinoid-based medications in the future.

And while some people see this as an indicator that federal legalization is not too far down the road, another reason some people believe legalization might finally be poised to happen is that the US federal government holds a patent on several cannabinoids, including CBD, as neuroprotectants, a blatant contradiction to the government's own insistence that cannabis has no known medicinal use. With this patent, the US Department of Health and Human Services has confirmed what many people have been advocating for decades, that cannabinoid medicine is real and offers wellness options that are otherwise not available.

In the meantime, knowing and understanding the basics of how and why cannabinoid-based medicine works is the main weapon any person can have against the tide of confusion surrounding hemp and hemp-derived CBD.

BOLD EXPLORERS
BLAZING THE TRAIL

I FOUND MY VOICE!

Those were the first words Robert said when we began talking about his experience with CBD. He was attending a rally at the Illinois State Capitol in January, 2016. The rally was being held to present the governor with petitions signed by thousands and thousands of people encouraging the state of Illinois to expand the number and variety of conditions allowing patients to qualify for a state medical marijuana card. Robert was surprised when he was unexpectedly asked to speak to the crowd about his condition, Rheumatoid Arthritis, and why it should be a qualifying condition.

He remembers it was a cold, overcast day. There was a large crowd gathered outside the capitol building, and many people honked and offered the "thumbs up" hand signal as they drove by, including ambulances and firetrucks. He felt they were offering their support for medical marijuana as a safe alternative to opioids, which were claiming the lives of too many people, but the ambulances and firetrucks had never needed to respond to emergencies involving medical marijuana.

Not only surprised when he was asked to speak, he was terrified. Generally, he was a shy and quiet man. He was so nervous to speak in front of the crowd that he doesn't even remember what he said. But he did it! He remembers the crowd responding to him in a positive way, so apparently, he did a good job.

Sadly, he also remembers the governor didn't even come out to address the crowd that was gathered. Rather than come outside to accept the petitions, he sent his aide, who unceremoniously collected them, then turned around and went right back inside.

But Robert had found his voice! At the time, he was regularly attending information/education sessions about the health benefits of medical marijuana. The sessions were being held at his local public library.

Life has a way of throwing curve balls, and when he found himself unexpectedly returning to his childhood home in Iowa, he used the same strategy to offer information/education sessions about Cannabis Medicine at the local public library in his hometown. His very first session in Iowa, held in 2016, had a total of 12 people show up, and three of them were family members. But just two short years later, in 2018, his information/education sessions had an audience of 40 people for the medical marijuana sessions and 30 for his sessions about hemp and hemp-derived CBD.

Robert says the more he learned, the better off he was, and he continues learning as much as he can about Cannabis Medicine. He remains dedicated to raising awareness about the benefits of Cannabis Medicine.

Robert was involved in an accident in 1994 that shattered his tibial plateau, or the top of his tibia. He went through a series of operations to help correct the damage, and he is able to walk. But he has a lot of pain. Especially on cold days, and days when the weather is changing. He's used a variety of options to try to manage the pain, but he gets the best results from a combination of oral CBD drops and rubbing CBD salve on his painful knee. He also uses the salve for inflammation from his Rheumatoid Arthritis, and gets a positive result from that, as well. But his greatest benefit from using the CBD oil is how it has supported his sobriety. The CBD has helped curb his cravings. He's currently gone seven months without a drink, and is looking forward to many more!

Having found his voice by speaking about Cannabis Medicine, Robert has also used his newfound voice for other purposes. He is an avid advocate against unfair circumstances in the workplace, and more recently in politics.

Keep up the good work, Robert! You are an inspiration!

PART
Two

"Nature itself is the best physician."

—HIPPOCRATES

THIS SECTION INCLUDES some fairly dense science about how and why Cannabis Medicine works. We have included this information because we think it is important.

And it's a good read!!!!!

However, if there is more information here than you really want or need, please feel free to go directly to Chapter 5 to read the chapter by a pioneering Cannabis Medicine doctor.

Chapter

3

FOR TENS OF THOUSANDS OF YEARS, humans have been involved in an ongoing clinical trial with medicinal plants. We have used plants as medicine as long as we've existed. Ancient cultures successfully met all their needs with the natural resources in their area, including plants. They developed well-stocked pharmacies made up of roots, leaves, flowers, and even trees. Full of beauty and sustenance, the natural world offered healing potential for those who knew what to look for and where to look. Archeological excavations dated as far back as 60,000 years ago have found remains of plants, including cannabis, were being used for medicinal purposes.

Ancient societies considered plant medicine a delicate magic. Throughout much of history, humans believed the "vital spirit" of a plant was an essential element of its medicinal effects. Plant medicines were believed to heal the soul, mind, and body. Then in the early 1800s, scientists successfully isolated morphine from opium, leading to the idea of single, non-living compounds in the chemistry of plants as the source of their healing qualities. This philosophical shift led to the model in place today where plants are basically seen simply as resources that generate chemicals. Over time, scientists decided actual plants were not even necessary to produce medications, because chemists could synthesize compounds that were more potent (though, obviously, more toxic!) than the natural products Mother Nature provided.

In the early 20th century, there really weren't very many effective medications, but the few available were plant-based. For example, there was aspirin made from willow bark, digoxin made from foxglove, quinine made from cinchona bark, and morphine made from poppies. Many conventional medications are actually products of plants, but do not use the entire plant.[35] Clearly this system cannot capture or explain the complex natural healing possibilities inherent in many plants. Just as humans cannot be explained by simply reducing us down to our component parts, the healing effects of plants cannot necessarily be reduced to single elements.

With a new passion for studying plants as medicine, scientists are beginning to understand scientific evidence supporting the idea that plants are often safer and more effective than traditional medicines, especially for chronic diseases.[36] Medical schools and schools of pharmacy are reviving courses in science-based herbalism and medications made from plants, while schools of naturopathic and holistic medicine are more popular than ever. And the increasing acceptance of botanical medicine is likely to continue. When botanical medicines are used carefully, based on compelling scientific evidence and sound therapeutic practice, then they can and should have a place in modern medicine.[37]

And they certainly do! Between 1990 and 1997, the use of botanical medicines increased by 380 percent in the United States.[38] Additionally, the World Health Organization reports 75 to 85 percent of the world's population rely on botanical medicine dispensed by traditional healers for their primary healthcare.[39] By 2010, the global retail sale of botanical dietary supplements amounted to more than $25 billion, according to *Nutraceuticals World*.[40]

Herbal medicine and traditional western medicine have several important differences. For one thing, herbal medicine practitioners generally believe whole plant remedies offer greater effects than the sum total of the individual compounds, so they use unpurified plant extracts with multiple elements. They also claim toxicity is reduced with whole plants. Although any two samples of a particular herbal medication might have slightly different proportions of the main compounds, herbal practitioners say this usually does not cause clinical problems or affect results. In laboratory settings, plant extracts have been shown to have anti-inflammatory, vasodilatory, antimicrobial, anticonvulsant, sedative, antipyretic effects, and other healing qualities.[41]

THE ENTOURAGE EFFECT

Research into the medicinal effects of CBD has shown it is effective for an ever-expanding list of health issues, but pure CBD extracts do not necessarily provide the best results. A growing body of research shows CBD offers the best results when it is taken in combination with the full range of other chemical compounds in cannabis plants. This theoretical principle, known as "The Entourage Effect," states that when all of the multiple compounds inherent in cannabis plants work together, their medicinal effects are enhanced. The group dynamic of the entourage effect creates dramatic properties that do not exist with pure CBD.

Health benefits from CBD seem limitless when using full-spectrum products made from high-quality hemp, and the entourage effect is one of the reasons why. The entourage effect means CBD is not the only chemical compound responsible for the results it produces; other compounds in hemp strengthen the effects of the CBD. With the entourage effect, no single chemical element in hemp, including CBD, is considered the most important. Rather, each compound plays an important role, so if any component is missing, the total overarching effect is compromised.

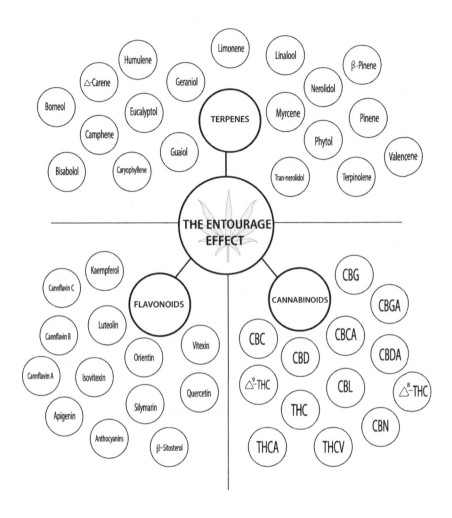

With the entourage effect, hundreds of different compounds in hemp interact with each other simultaneously to create the total effect. In order to benefit from the entourage effect, CBD must be taken as either full-spectrum or broad-spectrum hemp extract because it contains the complete range of hemp's natural phytochemicals, including trace amounts of THC. Cannabinoids like CBD are influenced by the presence of compounds like terpenes and flavonoids, plus lipids and nutritional components like omega acids. With multiple compounds working together, their medicinal effects are all enhanced.

Most of the research into the entourage effect has focused on the interactions between THC and CBD. For example, researchers reviewed a 2010 clinical trial involving the pain reliever Sativex, which is prescribed in several countries for patients living with multiple sclerosis, though Sativex has not been approved by the FDA, so it is not available to MS patients living in the US. Sativex includes a 1:1 mixture of THC and CBD.

Through a controlled study, Sativex was given to people experiencing severe pain associated with cancer. Some of the participants were given Sativex, some were given a preparation of pure THC extract, and others were given a placebo. Sativex was found to offer a significant pain-killing effect in 40 percent of the patients who took it, making it twice as effective as the pure THC extract, even though the amount of THC in both preparations was the same. This can only mean the CBD enhanced the pain-fighting potency of the THC. Further research showed Sativex does not cause the kinds of side effects often experienced with pure THC.[42]

Another study from 2016 compared the experiences of people who smoked pure THC with those of people who smoked cannabis products with both THC and CBD. Those who smoked the pure THC had memory problems and other cognitive difficulties, while those who smoked the products with blended THC and CBD did not.[43]

One exciting area of medicinal promise related to the entourage effect is learning and understanding how cannabinoids and terpenes work together to strengthen their healing qualities. Research into the effects created by combinations of cannabinoids and terpenes is truly limited, but a 2018 meta-analysis showed pure CBD extracts were far less effective at reducing the number of seizures epilepsy patients had compared to extracts that blended CBD with other cannabinoids and terpenes. 71% of those who took the blended preparation had fewer seizures, while only 46% of those who used the pure CBD had similar results. These results emphasize the significance of the entourage effect.[44]

As research continues and scientists expand their knowledge and understanding of how the chemical compounds in hemp work together, we can anticipate them being able to offer different ways of working with the entire range of compounds in hemp to enhance and expand the full range of medicinal effects.

FLAVONOIDS

As research into the ways various chemical compounds in cannabis plants work together continues, scientists are recognizing the importance flavonoids bring to the entourage effect. Known to regulate the cellular cycle -- the ordered events when a cell is getting ready to divide – flavonoids also attract pollinators and protect plants from diseases, pests, and fungi; plus, they filter UV rays. Flavonoids are found in every flower, fruit, and vegetable. They are a group of plant metabolites that provide health benefits through cell signaling pathways between cannabinoids and terpenes.

As researchers continue analyzing the effects flavonoids add to the medicinal qualities of cannabis, they are finding these compounds, both on their own and in concert with other compounds, have healing qualities including antioxidant, anti-inflammatory, anti-allergic, antibiotic, and antidiarrheal. Certain flavonoids even protect the genome from chemical carcinogens, or cancer-causing compounds. Approximately 6,000 flavonoids have been identified, and they are organized into six categories:[45]

Flavones: Colorless crystalline compounds serving as the basis of a number of white or yellow plant pigments, these compounds are the subject of increasing interest because of their biological activities. Flavones are associated with overall antioxidant benefits.[46]

Anthocyanidins: Found naturally in a number of foods, anthocyanidins are the pigments that give red, purple, and blue plants their color. In addition to acting as antioxidants and fighting free radicals, anthocyanidins provide anti-inflammatory, anti-viral, and anti-carcinogenic benefits. Anthocyanidins are associated with heart health and antioxidant effects, plus they help prevent diabetes and obesity.[47]

Flavonones: A small group of polyphenols found specifically in citrus fruits, flavonones are aromatic, colorless ketones associated with cardiovascular health and relaxation, plus overall antioxidant and anti-inflammatory activity.[48]

Isoflavones: These compounds are phytoestrogens, meaning they are plant compounds with qualities that mimic the hormone estrogen. Isoflavones are highly concentrated in soybeans and soy products, as well as legumes. Research suggests they may be beneficial in lowering risks for hormonal cancers, like breast, endometrial, and prostate cancers; they are also being studied as a way to help with menopausal symptoms.[49]

Flavanols: There are three primary types of flavanols -
• catechins
• dimers
• polymers
  Catechins are useful in relieving symptoms of chronic fatigue syndrome, and they are associated with cardiovascular and neurologic health. Also associated with strong anti-inflammatory and antioxidant qualities leading to prevention of chronic disease, catechins are especially common in green and white teas, while dimers, which are associated with lowering cholesterol, are found in black tea.[50]

Flavan-3-ols: A group of bio-actives, or non-essential dietary components with significant impact on health, flavan-3-ols are found in a wide range of different foods, so they are one of the most commonly consumed flavonoids. Flavan-3-ols improve hypertension, dyslipidemia (an abnormal level of cholesterol and other lipids), insulin resistance, and obesity.[51]

Numerous studies have shown dramatic health benefits from these phytonutrients. A published review of all flavonoid studies published over a period of eleven years reached the conclusion that a diet rich in flavonoids lowers the risk for several different cancers: anthocyanidins decrease the risk for lung cancer, while flavanols reduce the risk for prostate cancer. The best way to know you're getting an adequate supply of all six types of flavonoids is to eat a variety of fruits and vegetables, which offer the most well-rounded benefits.[52]

Flavonoids help regulate cellular activity and protect against oxidative stress caused by free radicals. They help the body function more efficiently and protect against everyday toxins and stressors. Flavonoids are also effective antioxidant agents, and a growing body of scientific research shows flavonoids play a beneficial role in disease prevention.[53]

Significant health benefits attributed to flavonoids include:

Longevity: A study involving more than 50,000 participants over a period of 2 decades found eating flavonoid-rich foods helps prevent disease and extend life. The study, published in 1995 in the journal *Archives of Internal Medicine*, concluded, "[W]e provide evidence that an achievable dietary intake of total and individual flavonoid subclasses is associated with a lower risk of all causes for cardio-vascular-disease-related, and cancer-related mortality." The study looked at men across seven countries and found eating flavonoids was clearly associated with longevity, and eating flavonoids could account for 25 percent of the observed difference in mortality rates from both coronary heart disease and cancer.[54]

Weight management: Flavonoids are also associated with inflammation and weight loss. They can decrease the levels of an appetite-suppressing hormone, leptin, which helps inhibit hunger and regulate energy balance, playing an important role in food consumption.[55]

A study published in the *British Medical Journal* reported that in a group of 124,000 men and women over a period of 25 years, participants who indicated higher consumption of a variety of flavonoids were less likely to gain weight than those who consumed foods with lower or no flavonoids. The researchers accounted for differences in lifestyle variables such as smoking, physical activity levels, and other dietary factors in order to isolate the impact of the flavonoids.[56]

Cardiovascular disease prevention: Because of their antioxidant and anti-inflammatory behaviors, flavonoids are associated with cardiovascular disease prevention. According to the website *George Mateljan Foundation's World's Healthiest Foods* flavonoids lower the risk of atherosclerosis by protecting LDL cholesterol from free radical damage. They also improve the quality of blood vessel walls.[57]

Several studies have found an association between increased flavonoid intake and decreased risk for cardiovascular disease across various groups, including postmenopausal women, male smokers, and middle-age men and women. One study of more than 10,000 men and women, published in 2002 in the *American Journal of Clinical Nutrition*, found those with higher levels of quercetin had lower rates of ischemic heart disease, and those with higher levels of kaempferol, naringenin, and hesperetin had lower cerebrovascular disease rates. According to the *Linus Pauling Institute*, various flavonoids, including quercetin, are known to be effective at preventing platelet accumulation, which contributes to heart disease because blood clots can lead to strokes and other problems.[58]

Diabetes prevention: Flavonoids are helpful with preventing and managing diabetes. Different classes of flavonoids have been connected to limiting the impacts of diabetic complications like neuropathy and retinopathy, while other studies have shown promise in using flavonoid supplements to help manage diabetes. Regarding diabetes prevention, flavonoids, especially anthocyanidins and flavones, have been connected to inhibiting insulin resistance and lowering diabetes risk.[59]

A study published in 2013 in the journal *Diabetic Medicine* found that among men with type 2 diabetes, adding a flavonoid-rich spice mix made up of rosemary, garlic, ginger, black pepper, and oregano to hamburger meat significantly improved their vascular function.[60]

Cancer prevention: According to the *Linus Pauling Institute*, animal studies with flavonoids have shown positive results with regard to lung, mouth, stomach, colon, skin, and other cancers.[61]

The most promising studies using humans are with breast and stomach cancer. A large study published in 2003 in the *British Journal of Cancer* found that women with higher levels of flavone intake had a lower risk for developing breast cancer,[62] while a study in *Cancer Causes & Control* found a correlation between kaempferol intake and reduced risk for gastric cancer.[63]

Neurodegenerative disease prevention: Flavonoids' anti-inflammatory and antioxidant effects help protect against neurodegenerative diseases like Alzheimer's and Parkinson's. A large-scale study published in 2000 in the *European Journal of Epidemiology* found, among elderly men and women, those with the highest levels of flavonoids had a 50% lower risk of developing dementia over the next five years than those with the lowest levels of flavonoids.[64]

According to *World's Healthiest Foods*, flavonoids also increase blood flow to the brain, improving cognitive function.[65] A study published in 2007 in the *American Journal of Epidemiology* found that elderly men and women with higher flavonoid intake had better cognitive performance at the start of the study, and significantly less age-related cognitive decline over the next 10 years than those with lower flavonoid intake.[66]

Management of Chronic Pain and Inflammation: Flavonoids are potent antioxidants with the potential to minimize tissue damage, and to have beneficial properties with inflammatory diseases. They act on different peripheral neuropathic pain conditions by blocking oxidative stress, activating glial cells, and mitochondrial dysfunction.[67]

Another medical review evaluated the anti-inflammatory and pain-relieving properties of flavonoids. These studies show flavonoids reduce the cellular response to pain. Researchers believe flavonoids could be used to help manage chronic pain and inflammatory diseases.[68]

Use with Viral Infections: Numerous laboratory studies have shown that certain flavonoids prevent cell replication of viruses including H1N1 flu, HIV, SARS, and RSV.[69]

CONSUMING FLAVONOIDS

Eating a diet with a variety of fresh fruits and vegetables is the best way to know you're getting adequate flavonoids, plus there are no side effects from eating plant-based foods. In addition, many types of flavonoids are available in supplement form, providing an option for people who struggle to get enough fruits and vegetables in their diet. However, the *Linus Pauling Institute* notes that quercetin supplements can cause headaches, tingling in the arms and legs, and very high doses can cause kidney damage.[70]

FLAVONOIDS AND CANNABIS

People usually think the flavors and aromas of cannabis are due to terpenes, which is not untrue. But flavonoids also play an important role in creating the distinct characteristics between different strains, which are the result of the synergistic qualities exchanged when flavonoids and terpenes interact. Also, the pigmentation of purple cannabis plants is the result of flavonoids known as anthoxanthins or anthocyanidins.

There are twenty-three flavonoids unique to cannabis plants, known as cannaflavins. They work in conjunction with terpenes and other flavonoids to create the unique tastes, aromas, and pigmentations specific to individual strains. In 1986, Marilyn Barrett, a researcher from the University of London, successfully isolated two cannaflavins and found the anti-inflammatory effects produced by Cannaflavin A and Cannaflavin B are up to 30x more potent than those produced by Aspirin. However, the amount of cannaflavins in cannabis is actually very small, making up less than 0.15% of the fresh weight of cannabis, meaning massive amounts of cannabis would have to be consumed in order for these effects to be accomplished. In order to sidestep this issue, researchers have begun to engineer cannaflavins separately from the cannabis plant. By successfully identifying the genes in cannabis responsible for producing canna-flavins, researchers have been able to produce them in isolation. Flavonoids could very well be the next big thing in medical cannabis science.[71]

The most common cannaflavins, along with their known health benefits, are:

- **Cannaflavin A**: Studies show it has anti-inflammatory properties stronger than those in Aspirin.[72]
- **Cannaflavin B**: Works particularly well against pancreatic cancer, one of the deadliest cancers with only a dismal 8% survival rate.[73]
- **Cannflavin A and Cannflavin B**: are more effective with pain relief than either THC or CBD.[74]
- **Cannaflavin C**: Has anti-inflammatory, anti-fungal, antioxidant, and anti-carcinogenic potential.[75]
- **Quercetin**: Has medicinal qualities including pain relief, anti-inflammatory, cardioprotective, anticarcinogenic, immuno-protective, and it eases skin irritations when used topically.[76]
- **Luteolin**: Has numerous useful actions, including anti-oxidant, anti-inflammatory, microglia inhibition, neuroprotection, and it is helpful with increasing memory.[77]
- **Naringin**: Displays strong anti-inflammatory and antioxidant activities; several studies suggest naringin is beneficial for helping with obesity, diabetes, hypertension, and metabolic syndrome.[78]
- **Butin**: Reduces oxidative stress-related cell dysfunction and cell death.[79]
- **Hesperetin**: Benefits cardiovascular function, type 2 diabetes, and anti-inflammation.[80] Additionally, hesperitin is beneficial for cutaneous (skin) functions, including wound healing, UV protection, anti-inflammation, antimicrobial, skin cancer prevention, and skin lightening.[81]
- **Orientin**: Has medicinal properties including antioxidant, antiaging, antiviral, antibacterial, anti-inflammation, vasodilatation and cardioprotective, radiation protective, neuroprotective, antidepressant, anti-adipogenesis, and antinociceptive effects.[82]

- **Taxifolin**: Helps manage inflammation, tumors, microbial infections, oxidative stress, cardiovascular and liver disorders.[83]
- **Aromadendrin**: Has anti-oxidant, anti-proliferation, and anti-inflammatory properties, plus it is a potential medicine for type 2 diabetes and cardiovascular diseases.[84]
- **Catechins**: Are natural antioxidants that help prevent cell damage and reduce the formation of free radicals in the body, protecting cells and molecules from damage. Their medicinal qualities include anti-inflammatory, antioxidant, and help lowering cholesterol.[85]
- **Vitexin and Isovitexin**: Are antioxidant, anti-inflammatory, anti-cancer, antidiabetic, neuroprotective, and antinociceptive.[86]

As scientists and researchers continue learning about the health benefits of flavonoids, and particularly cannaflavins, more studies are definitely on the horizon. The puzzle of how the various medicinal elements of cannabis work together remains challenging, but slowly the pieces are being fit together, and the picture they are beginning to present is exciting. We look forward to a future when all the therapeutic compounds in cannabis will be fully understood and appreciated, and embraced for the medicinal benefits they offer. In the meantime, one thing is obvious: with the kinds of health benefits already identified, we should all be eating plenty of fresh fruits and vegetables!

TERPENES

A set of chemical elements in cannabis that have received considerably more attention than flavonoids, terpenes are organic compounds that help make up the aromas and flavors in plants. Terpenes are the reason that pine trees smell like pine, and that flowers, fruits, and vegetables come in such a broad spectrum of colors. Also found in spices, teas, and essential oils, terpenes (along with flavonoids) are responsible for the aromas, flavors, and pigmentations that distinguish one cannabis strain from another.

Traditionally, terpenes have been considered important for their therapeutic and medicinal qualities, and individual strains of hemp are bred with specific combinations and ratios of terpenes to accomplish specific effects in CBD formulations.

Cannabis is known to have over 100 different terpenes; they bring therapeutic value to hemp and/or marijuana according to their particular medicinal properties interacting with other compounds in the plants, especially cannabinoids. Terpenes are known to help with pain, inflammation, depression, anxiety, addiction, epilepsy, cancer, fungal and bacterial infections, and much more. Testing for terpene content is a standard test performed by analytical labs who then report it in the COA, so savvy consumers will have a better idea of the specific effects a strain is likely to have, depending on its terpene content.

The concept of terpenes directly impacting brain function seems obvious today, but for many years people had a difficult time distinguishing between the direct effects of terpenes on brain function and their indirect effects on mood. Today, we understand terpenes directly affect brain processes by modulating the behavior of brain cells. For example, we know the sense of smell is linked to centers in the brain where the complex activities of emotion and memory occur, and these centers are stimulated by scents generated by terpenes.

As the idea of the entourage effect continues gaining acceptance, researchers are paying more attention to terpenes. According to the entourage effect, cannabis' therapeutic benefits are enhanced by each chemical compound of the plant working in cooperation with the full array of other compounds, including cannabinoids and terpenes, rather than any single compound's effect on its own, including CBD. This idea suggests terpenes modulate the effects of specific cannabinoids. Each strain of hemp has a unique combination of terpenes that alters the way cannabinoids interact with the receptors of the Endocannabinoid system. They influence the effects of cannabinoids, strengthening the medicinal benefits of the hemp.

But the entourage effect does not mean terpenes don't have direct actions themselves. There are hundreds of terpenes in cannabis plants, but a few stand out as being medicinally significant. Here are some facts about the 8 most prominent terpenes in hemp:

- **MYRCENE:** One of the most common terpenes found in cannabis plants, myrcene represents between 30% and 65% of the essential oils extracted from the plant. Known for its earthy, musky aroma, myrcene supports relaxation and aids with sleep. Found in hops, lemongrass, parsley, and wild thyme, myrcene has been linked to enhanced transdermal absorption, potentially opening up another avenue for greater cannabinoid uptake. Myrcene has a long list of therapeutic benefits.

   Anti-inflammatory: A 2015 study published in the *European Journal of Pharmacology* used human cartilage cells to investigate myrcene's potential effects on osteoarthritis. The researchers found that myrcene had an anti-inflammatory influence on the cells, and that it slowed disease progression and the tissue damage associated with it.[87]

   Anti-tumor: A 2015 study published in the Journal of the *Korean Society for Applied Biological Chemistry* suggested that myrcene may play a role in encouraging anti-metastatic activity in human breast cancer cells. Because the study was performed on cells rather than directly on humans, more research is necessary to determine if myrcene could have a direct impact on killing malignant tumors in cancer patients, but the initial evidence is promising.[88]

   Sedative: A study published in 2002 in the journal *Phytomedicine* showed myrcene may have a sedative effect in mice at very high doses. Myrcene increased barbiturate sleeping time when compared to a control group, demonstrating the terpene's potential as a sedative.[89]

Antioxidant: Myrcene may have the ability to protect against ultra-violet light-induced aging in human skin, according to a 2017 study published in the *American Journal of Chinese Medicine*. By acting partially as an antioxidant, myrcene may very well be a beneficial additive to anti-aging and sunscreen lotions. As the most frequently encountered terpene in cannabis, myrcene may offer hope for those coping with osteoarthritis and other inflammatory conditions. [90]

* **CARYOPHYLLENE**: Another common terpene in cannabis plants, caryophyllene is easy to recognize by its spicy, pepper-like aroma and taste. Caryophyllene is the only known terpene that displays characteristics of a cannabinoid by interacting directly with CB2 receptors in the ECS. Its medicinal properties include:

Anti-inflammatory: With measurable anti-inflammatory proper-ties, caryophyllene potentially has the ability to help with anxiety and depression, plus its strong anti-inflammatory qualities make it a possible therapy for inflammatory bowel disease since it binds with CB2 receptors.

Other medicinal qualities: Caryophyllene is widely believed to provide digestive protection, pain relief, and antibacterial activity. Many consumers report that using cannabis strains rich in caryo-phyllene facilitates a sense of calm in the gut, which could aid in anxiety-related issues and support a feeling of general wellbeing. Plus, caryophyllene shows promise in reducing alcohol-induced cravings.

Also called beta-caryophyllene or BCP, this terpene can be found in aromatic oils like rosemary and clove oil, and is commonly found in hops, cloves, black pepper, oregano, cinnamon, and basil. Caryophyllene is a bigger molecule than other terpenes like myrcene, so caryophyllene's molecular structure also contains a cyclobutane ring, which is extremely rare in nature and is not found in any other known cannabis terpene.[91]

- **LINALOOL**: Most commonly linked with lavender, linalool is a major terpene in many different cannabis strains; it has a floral scent that also suggests a hint of spice. Linalool's therapeutic properties include:

Pain Relief: Linalool helps moderate pain and inflammation by interacting with the central nervous system, helping regulate the production and absorption of brain chemicals like adenosine and glutamate. In one study, patients who had undergone gastric banding surgery found that linalool helped decrease their reliance on opioid painkillers. Also, when used in conjunction with morphine, inhaling linalool has been shown to help decrease the amount of morphine patients need following surgery.[92]

Anti-inflammatory: Linalool reduces the excitability of spinal cord cells that transmit pain signals to the brain and increases levels of a central nervous system depressant, helping with pain relief and sleep.[93]

Therapy for Alzheimer's disease: Linalool was administered to mice with three mutations associated with familial Alzheimer's disease showed improved learning, spatial memory, and greater risk assessment behavior in a study with an elevated plus maze, leading researchers to believe linalool could slow and even reverse some of the cognitive impairments associated with Alzheimer's disease.[94]

Anti-Microbial: A study demonstrated that linalool has the potential to fight infections naturally, an important quality considering current issues with drug-resistant microbes.[95]

Other medicinal qualities: Linalool is thought to support the immune system and promote restful sleep, and it has been used in traditional medicine practices for its sedative and anti-epileptic properties.[96]

• **PINENE**: Named for its scent, pinene smells like pine trees, but it is also found in conifer trees, orange peels, turpentine, rosemary, dill, basil, and parsley. There are two types of pinene, known as alpha-pinene and beta-pinene. Generally, alpha-pinene is the terpene referenced when discussing it in relation to cannabis. Research is still confirming pinene's medicinal effects and benefits, but the following uses are currently accepted:

Anti-inflammatory: Alpha-pinene has an anti-inflammatory effect, making it a potential candidate for use with certain inflammatory diseases.[97]

Bronchodilator: Pinene has a comforting effect on airways and bronchial passages. Though it seems contradictory, using cannabis that has a high pinene content with a vape pen or vaporizer can help calm inflammatory responses like asthma.[98]

Anti-anxiety: Mice that underwent chronic inhalation (90 minutes per day) of alpha pinene over a five-day period demonstrated anti-anxiety effects.[99]

Pain relief: Alpha-pinene is ideal for people who like to use marijuana for chronic pain but don't want the adverse effects on short-term memory.

The pain-relieving properties of pinene have been demonstrated in preclinical studies (animal or cell cultures only, not humans).

- Frankincense which was pinene-dominant produced higher anti-inflammatory and anti-analgesic effects than water in a mouse model.
- Pinene has been shown to alleviate tooth pain in mice.[100]

May help ease short-term memory impairment associated with THC: Pinene supports memory and improves focus by providing a concentration boost and feelings of alertness.[101]

- **HUMULENE**: Humulene has been used for centuries in holistic Eastern medical practices. Its subtle aroma is earthy and woody with spicy herbal notes. Humulene is found in coriander, basil, clove, black pepper, sage, and balsam fir trees. The medical and therapeutic potential of humulene is expansive and well-researched, and include:

Anticancer: Humulene is believed to be an active mechanism in fighting tumors, evidenced by its ability to produce Reactive Oxygen Species (ROS). A 2016 study showed that, when combined with cannabinoids and other terpenes, it may help terminate cancer cells.[102]

Antibacterial: In another study, humulene was shown to have antibacterial properties, proving to be active against the bacterium Staphylococcus aureus (golden staph).[103]

Anti-inflammatory: Humulene's anti-inflammatory qualities are so strong that it has been compared to the steroid dexamethasone, which is listed as one of the WHO's most essential medicines; it is effective with arthritis, bursitis, fibromyalgia, and other conditions that benefit from reducing inflammation.[104]

Other medicinal qualities: Humulene plays a role in pharmacokinetics, the study of how human bodies absorb, distribute, metabolize, and excrete medications. So far, it appears to be distributed quickly throughout the body with both oral and topical absorption of an oil from the tropical plant black sage, which has anti-inflammatory, antifungal, and antibacterial properties.[105]

- **LIMONENE**: Limonene is the second most abundant terpene in nature. Used in commercial food flavorings, cosmetics, fragrances, and cleaning products, Limonene is also popular with people who practice aromatherapy. A stress-reliever and mood enhancer, it improves absorption of other terpenes and chemicals through skin, mucous membranes, and the digestive tract. Limonene is found in oranges, rosemary, juniper, peppermint, and a variety of fruit rinds. Researchers and scientists actually know very little about how limonene works in the brain and body, and how much is needed to achieve the benefits. In many of the limonene studies, high doses were used; considerably higher than the amounts found in cannabis, proving more cannabis-focused research is needed. So far, studies on limonene have shown potential in the following applications:

Elevated mood: Anxiety and depression are associated with low levels of neurotransmitters, the chemicals that transfer information from one nerve cell to another, including serotonin and dopamine. Stress-reducing chemicals transmitted through the nervous system, serotonin works on emotional processing, while dopamine is associated with pleasurable feelings. In a 2013 study, limonene was found to increase serotonin and decrease anxiety-related symptoms. Limonene also affects adenosine receptors, triggering increased release of dopamine. Because of the connection between anxiety and depression, researchers suggest it can be helpful for both conditions.[106]

Stress relief: Several studies show limonene's stress-relieving properties. As far back as 1955, 9 of 15 patients who used limonene showed a decrease in their need for antidepressant medication and an increase in immune system functioning plus normalization of stress hormone levels.[107]

Help relieving heartburn and gastric reflux: Limonene has been used clinically to dissolve cholesterol-containing gallstones. Because of its gastric acid neutralizing effect and its support of normal peristalsis, it has also been used to relieve heartburn and gastroesophageal reflux (GERD).[108]

- **OCIMENE:** The scent produced by ocimene is often described as sweet, herbal, and woody. Additionally, ocimene is said to have undertones of citrus. Ocimene occurs naturally in allspice, mint, parsley, marjoram, tarragon, bay laurel, basil, pepper, and mangoes. Like other terpenes, ocimene helps these plants defend themselves from pests and disease. Remarkably, research indicates that when a plant is being attacked by insect pests, it releases ocimene to deter the pests and to "warn" other plants nearby about the problem. A study suggests ocimene may have anti-convulsant properties that could help prevent seizures.

Decongestant: Ocimene helps clear airways and improve breathing when smoked or vaped.[109]

Anti-fungal: Plants with high levels of ocimene are traditionally used as preservatives to extend the shelf life of dairy products in certain parts of the world. Research has shown tarragon, a plant with very high ocimene levels, has anti-bacterial and anti-fungal properties, giving it the ability to reduce food spoiling. Additional research shows ocimene effectively inhibits the Candida albicans fungus and works as an insecticide against some pests.[110]

Anti-viral: Research indicates that the oil of plants containing high levels of ocimene inhibit the SARS virus.[111]

- **TERPINOLENE**: The least-common among the "common terpenes," terpinolene is present in plenty of cannabis strains, though usually in small amounts. Terpinolene's aroma is more multidimensional than some of the other terpenes in cannabis; it is piney, floral, herbaceous, and even a little citrusy. Like most terpenes, terpinolene isn't unique to cannabis; it also shows up in lilacs, tea tree, nutmeg, cumin, and apples.

Antifungal: Terpinolene has antifungal effects on conditions like toenail fungus and ringworm.[112]

Antioxidant: A 2015 study showed that low doses of terpinolene have antioxidant properties without harming lymphocytes. Another study showed that it prevents oxidation of LDL cholesterol, so terpinolene likely has heart health benefits.[113]

Sedative: Terpinolene is known for its sedative properties, which are recommended for anxiety and insomnia. When mixed with lavender and lilac, terpinolene is used for certain sleep disorders.[114]

Anti-Cancer: A 2013 study found that terpinolene may be a strong antiproliferative agent for brain tumor cells, indicating terpinolene may protect against inflammation and oxidative damage, both associated with cancer.[115]

These eight terpenes represent the ones most prominent in cannabis, but there are numerous others, supporting the idea of the entourage effect. Like the ones included here, many of the others have been studied for their individual medicinal qualities, yet many of them have not had the benefit of such in-depth analysis.

The specific ratio and composition of terpenes in cannabis strains are based on a variety of factors, including genetics, so identifying terpenes in cannabis and how they are constituted can play an instrumental role in establishing medical benefits between strains. More than 120 specific terpene compounds have been identified in cannabis plants, and every strain is made up of a unique type and composition. They are produced inside specialized hairs, called trichomes, located on the surface of the leaves and stems of plants. Terpenes are organic hydrocarbons that make up a major component of the plant's sticky resin, and they are produced by the same glands that produce cannabinoids.

Terpenes cause a variety of physiological processes and chemical responses, depending on specific strain combinations. In cannabis, they are not only the reason for its fragrance and color, but they work in conjunction with other chemical compounds like cannabinoids to produce specific effects.

Strain genetics, as well as cultivation methods, affect the types and amounts of terpenes found in specific hemp strains, and therefore the CBD products made from those strains.

CANNABINOIDS

Flavonoids and terpenes bring amazing medicinal properties to hemp, both individually and through the entourage effect. However, other chemical compounds in cannabis plants, known as cannabinoids, have the greatest medicinal effects because they interact directly with the nervous system and various organs in the human body. Cannabinoids are chemical compounds produced naturally by human bodies and by cannabis plants. The health benefits of cannabinoids are numerous: pain management, stress management, appetite control, energy metabolism, cardiovascular function, reward and motivation, reproduction, and sleep are just a few of the body's functions that cannabinoids impact. Research into the health benefits of cannabinoids like CBD is at an all-time high, opening up more possibilities for additional uses, and people are excited about the results.

Human bodies and cannabis plants both produce cannabinoids, so there are two types:

1. Endocannabinoids, also called endogenous cannabinoids, are molecules produced in and by the human body.

2. Phytocannabinoids are naturally occurring chemical compounds produced in and by plants, especially cannabis plants.

At least 480 different chemical compounds have been identified in cannabis, and among them are at least 113 cannabinoids. Like terpenes, phytocannabinoids are produced by glandular trichomes and concentrated in a sticky resin produced by cannabis plants.

When phytocannabinoids are introduced into the body, whether inhaled, ingested, or used topically, these compounds interact with cannabinoid receptors in what is known as the Endocannabinoid System (ECS). The ECS is discussed at length and in detail in the next chapter, so for now, just know different cannabinoids cause different effects depending on the type and location of the receptors they interact with. Because human bodies use cannabinoid molecules to regulate numerous bodily functions, they naturally have plentiful targets for phytocannabinoids.

Cannabinoids, whether endocannabinoids or phytocannabinoids, interact with receptors the way a key interacts with a lock. Cannabinoids, as the key, bind with receptors containing metabolic enzymes that break down the cannabinoids, unlocking their effects. Scientists have identified two main endocannabinoids so far, and two main cannabinoid receptors, though research indicates there are probably more of each.

Every function a human body performs relies on a delicate balance of factors, called homeostasis, in order to accomplish peak performance. Throughout the body, cannabinoids interacting with receptors set homeostatic responses into motion. Cannabinoids regulate every bodily function. The effects created by cannabinoids depend on the area of the brain or body involved. For example, in human brains, cannabinoid effects on the limbic system are known to affect memory, cognition, and psychomotor performance, while cannabinoid effects on the mesolimbic pathway influence reward and pleasure responses, plus they alter pain perception.

Millions of patients around the world are gaining access to solutions for conditions that were previously considered untreatable now that researchers are developing increased understanding of phytocannabinoids and their relationship with the human body. But cannabis is a complex plant and scientists don't always agree about how it affects the body. As cannabis research and medical applications continue to expand, it is critically important to remember that each person's endocannabinoid system is unique, so one person's body might have a different response to certain specific phytocannabinoids than somebody else's.[116]

PHYTOCANNABINOIDS

Phytocannabinoids, the ones produced by plants, cover the surface of cannabis plants as a defense mechanism to protect against environmental hazards like insects and harsh weather conditions, among other things. Interestingly, some other plants also produce these chemical compounds that interact with cannabinoid receptors. For example, cacao is rich in anandamide, the endogenous cannabinoid regulating mood, memory, appetite, and pain perception. Recently, researchers discovered black truffles are also rich in anandamide. Additionally, Kava, a medicinal tea from the Pacific islands, is rich in kavalactones, compounds that interact directly with cannabinoid receptors, which is probably why kava has a long-standing reputation as a natural remedy for both anxiety and pain.

Neither of the most famous cannabinoids, THC and CBD, are directly produced by cannabis plants. Rather, the plants synthesize cannabinoid acids which must be "activated" (decarboxylated), usually by heat, in order to produce either THC or CBD. Several related cannabinoid acids (identified by the initial A) are produced by cannabis, with THC-A and CBD-A the most abundant cannabinoids in most cannabis plants. Others have dramatically lower levels. When cannabinoid acids are exposed to heat energy, they lose their acidity and become neutral. Through decarboxylation (heating), each cannabinoid acid evolves into its corresponding phytocannabinoid. The cannabinoid acids don't cause intoxication, but they do have a variety of therapeutic qualities very similar to those of flavonoids and terpenes.[117]

DECARBOXYLATION REACTION OF Δ^9 THC

THCA
$(C_{22}H_{30}O_4)$

THC
$(C_{21}H_{30}O_2)$

$+ CO_2$

HEAT > 105°C

Phytocannabinoids are not intoxicating themselves, but their presence has direct influence on the effects of THC. For example, CBD influences the way THC interacts with certain cannabinoid receptors. The quantity of cannabinoids a person takes can greatly influence how they will affect that person.

Another phytocannabinoid, THC-V, also influences THC's effects. Research suggests it may also cause some degree of intoxication, but that seems to depend on the amount taken. At relatively low doses, THC-V seems to block THC's ability to activate cannabinoid receptors, but at high doses, it activates them the same way THC does. One of the other phytocannabinoids that is not directly processed by cannabis is Cannabinol (CBN), a breakdown product of THC. Over time and with exposure to oxygen, THC gradually breaks down into CBN, which has anti-seizure, anti-inflammatory, and anti-biotic properties. Phytocannabinoids are separated into subclasses including:

- **Cannabigerols (CBG)**: bind to both receptors, where they strengthen the function of anandamide, the neurotransmitter that plays a role in enhancing pleasure and motivation. CBG also helps regulate appetite and sleep, and helps alleviate pain. [118]

- **Cannabichromenes (CBC)**: non-psychoactive cannabinoids that encourage the human brain to grow by increasing the viability of developing brain cells through a process known as neurogenesis.[119]

- **Cannabidiols (CBD)**: commonly used to address anxiety, and for patients who suffer through the misery of insomnia, studies suggest CBD may help with both falling asleep and staying asleep. CBD may also offer an option for helping with different types of chronic pain.[120]

- **Tetrahydrocannabinols (THC)**: the most promising uses for all forms of THC, including Delta 8 and Delta 10, which are currently receiving a lot of attention, are to counteract nausea associated with chemotherapy and to stimulate appetite.[121]

- **Cannabinol (CBN)**: created when THC-A oxidizes, CBN can be used effectively as a sleep aid or sedative; it has also been shown to help regulate the immune system and it works to relieve pain and inflammation caused by several conditions, including arthritis and Crohn's disease.[122]

- **Cannabicyclol (CBL)**: drastically understudied compared to THC and CBD; even lesser-known cannabinoids like CBG and CBN have been studied more than CBL, which is extremely difficult to extract from cannabis. However, one study showed CBL had virtually no effect on inhibiting production of prostaglandins, whereas every other cannabinoid tested did have inhibitory effects.[123]

- **Cannabielsoin (CBE)**: virtually nothing is known of CBE's beneficial or adverse effects. In one of the first studies assessing the formation of CBE, it was found CBE had little effect on inducing sleep or affecting body temperature in mice. CBE was also found to show negligible effects on inhibiting the human cytochrome, especially in comparison to CBD.[124]

- **Cannabitriol (CBT)**: there have been no studies on the benefits and adverse effects of CBT. However, in 2007, one study focused on the addictive effects of THC where researchers were looking for antibodies that could potentially mitigate the psychoactive components of THC. Their findings showed CBT was "the major degradation product of this reaction, demonstrating the ability of an antibody to catalyze a complex chemical transformation with therapeutic implications for helping with marijuana abuse." There are no other studies to confirm this finding, but if it is true, CBT is likely a non-psychoactive cannabinoid that, when present alongside THC, might diminish THC's psychoactive effects.[125]

- **Cannabivarin (CBV):** used in the care of psychiatric and mood disorders, brain tumors, neuropathic pain, and multiple sclerosis, CBV is also believed to have a positive impact on sexuality by increasing sexual desire. Appetite control, as well as regulation of metabolism and weight are also potential benefits of CBV. Additionally, research suggests this compound has a positive impact on sleep-wake cycles and could help with specific sleeping disorders. Furthermore, it is effective in reducing nausea and vomiting associated with chemotherapy.[126]

- **Tetrahydrocannabivarin (THCV):** relieves stress, plus it can help reduce or even prevent anxiety and panic attacks, so it plays an important role in easing the symptoms of post-traumatic-stress-disorder (PTSD).[127]

- **Cannabidivarin (CBDV):** significantly reduces the frequency and severity of seizures; it also reduces or even eliminates nausea, and helps reduce inflammation. CBDV is also beneficial for pain and mood disorders.[128]

- **Cannabichromevarin (CBCV):** an anti-inflammatory, antidepressant, antibiotic, analgesic, and antifungal. One particular area of interest regarding CBCV is easing seizures in children and infants.[129]

- **Cannabigerovarin (CBGV):** perceived to have no psychoactive effects, CBGV is considered "the mother of all cannabinoids" because it's a molecular precursor of major cannabinoids including THC and CBD. Research shows it enhances the competency of cellular receptors to bind with THC molecules. CBGV also enhances CBD metabolism, making CBD more powerful when paired with CBGV. It has painkilling and anti-inflammatory properties, making it effective at helping with conditions like fibromyalgia and arthritis. Furthermore, CBGV has been known to improve skin conditions. This cannabinoid is particularly useful for cancer patients undergoing chemotherapy and radiation because it is cytostatic in blood cancer cells, so it halts proliferation of cancer tissue.[130]

- **Cannabigerol Monoethyl Ether (CBGM)**: CBGM is being considered to potentially help patients with glaucoma, severe nausea, Crohn's disease, chronic pain, psoriasis, cancer, and arthritis.[131]

CLOSING THOUGHTS

Since our very beginnings, humans have been using plants as medicine. From the dawn of mankind, herbs and other plants have provided effective medicine for treating illnesses, and for promoting health and well-being. All plants have flavonoids and terpenes, which are known to have medicinal qualities, but the cannabis plant stands out among all other plants for its medicinal potential. Numerous cultures on every continent have used cannabis as medicine for eons.

Many of the flavonoids and terpenes in cannabis plants have tremendous medicinal qualities, and more are being identified regularly. The real medicinal promise of cannabis plants, though, lies with cannabinoids, chemical compounds remarkably similar to chemical compounds produced in and by human bodies to interact with receptors found on every single cell. Cannabinoids are being recognized as having significant medicinal qualities.

Our ancestors took specific natural remedies to fight or prevent specific illnesses. In that vein, there is a universal trend toward using herbal medications and other naturally-occurring products, so that many plants are enjoying a rebound after taking the back seat to modern medicine. Most conventional medications are chemically synthesized, though some are isolated from naturally occurring plants on the basis of their use in herbal medicine. Many people, seeking a more natural lifestyle as a path toward health, choose to use only herbal products; others use them in combination with traditional medications. The practice of herbal medicine uses more than 53,000 plant species, and sadly, many of them are facing the threat of extinction because of exploitation. Herbal medicines are an integral part of many cultures and geographical environments, and various herbal medicines have a unique way of treating diseases. In general, most herbal remedies are considered safe and well tolerated; they have been successfully used for thousands of years, both as food to promote health and as medicine to treat diseases.

Hope runs tremendously deep for the medicinal promise cannabinoids represent in terms of helping with chronic diseases and their debilitating symptoms. Research is barely out of the starting box for a variety of reasons, including the difficulties researchers have with accessing, handling, and studying cannabis. So far though, the limited results are absolutely exciting. We already know the ECS is instrumental in keeping internal processes stable. As researchers continue learning about how the ECS operates and exploring the possibilities this promising system offers through its interactions with cannabinoids, they will begin to map out the elusive path toward helping millions of people whose lives are affected by diseases and conditions currently considered untreatable.

BOLD EXPLORERS
BLAZING THE TRAIL

WE WERE CONTACTED BY A GENTLEMAN whose late wife put up one heck of a fight against Alzheimer's before finally succumbing to the disease. He wanted her story to be included in this book, but he felt strongly about protecting her privacy and anonymity, so we will simply call them John and Jane Doe.

As Jane's disease progressed, she struggled with anger – a situation that is not unusual for people living with Alzheimer's disease. When other efforts at managing her anger proved to be ineffective, John approached her doctor about the possibility of trying CBD. He had heard a little bit about its calming effects and thought it just might help her.

Jane's doctor wasn't knowledgeable about CBD, but indicated he would support John in having Jane trying it. John reports that shortly after starting on CBD therapy, Jane was definitely calmer. He said taking the CBD left her feeling more content and satisfied, less irritable and agitated. John reports, though, that the CBD seemed to help her in other ways, as well. He feels like she was able to do more with the CBD, that it helped her think more clearly and generally improved her quality of life. She took her CBD orally, and continued taking it for 3 or 4 years. With the help of the CBD, she was able to cut back on some of her other medications, including those that basically caused her to sleep as much as 20 – 22 hours per day. One medication that had this effect on her was her anti-seizure med, which made her "sleep all the time." John stated directly that he knows the CBD wasn't a cure of any sort, but he feels that once she started on the CBD, her lows weren't as low as they had been. He reports that her appetite improved, and she was eventually able to completely give up her seizure meds.

Jane's positive experience with CBD was an inspiration for another family member – an uncle of John's who was in his 70s and had always been absolutely skeptical about CBD and all Cannabis Medicine. He still considered all cannabis to be marijuana, and he had the attitude that medical marijuana programs and the CBD market were simply ways for "pot-heads" to exploit their interest in getting and staying stoned. However, as a cancer patient, he was taking "all kinds of medications," that came with the usual high incidence of side effects, so he decided to give CBD a try. He became a real believer in CBD therapy who said "it helped him a lot."

Chapter

4

THE MORE WE LEARN about the Endocannabinoid System (ECS), the more confused we are on a few different fronts. First of all, the system itself is complicated, and therefore confusing. Additionally, we are confused about how and why this amazing biological system is such a mystery to so many people. Why hasn't it made headline news? Why isn't it being taught, especially in medical schools? Discovered more than three decades ago, it remains unknown to most people.

Think about the amount of medical research that has been accomplished over the last 30 years: cancer research, AIDS research, mental illness research, just to start. The past 30 years have seen impressive advancements in the fight against many serious illnesses. But all of the mainstream medical research in the US has taken place without including research about the ECS in the picture.

Compared to the discovery of DNA in 1953, and the genetic code sequencing of RNA amino acids in 1961, which were both being taught in high school biology classes by the mid-1960s, the ECS has yet to make it into any significant number of classrooms. Excluding the ECS from science education at all levels, including medical schools, is the direct result of bad politics. Because hemp was classified with marijuana as a Schedule 1 Controlled Substance, there has been both a political inability and a systems-wide unwillingness to untie the promise of health benefits associated with cannabis in general, and CBD in particular, from the tangled web of the criminal justice system. Considering the ECS is the largest neurotransmitter system in the human brain and how the ECS plays an integral role in the operation of every other system in human bodies, combined with the medicinal potential of CBD and other cannabinoids, we are dumbstruck about why these aren't among the highest priorities in science and medicine education.

Considering that hemp-derived CBD is essentially legal at the federal level and, at the end of the year 2021, all but three states (Idaho, Nebraska, and Kansas) have some form of medical cannabis program, it is safe to say that Cannabis Medicine has become extremely popular. Whether dealing with injury or illness, more and more people are turning to Cannabis Medicine in addition to, or as an alternative to, traditional western medicine. In addition to the medicinal promise of cannabis, the ECS's effects on scavenging oxygen free radicals are applicable to all disease processes, so it has incredibly wide medical application. Doesn't that seem like it would be important for the next generation of medical professionals to know and understand? Medical schools are not keeping up with consumer demand and are not preparing future doctors to understand the true medicinal potential Cannabis Medicine presents. Medical students are not being trained to offer their patients professional recommendations about how to safely and effectively use CBD products.

An article published on November 1, 2017, summarized the results of a national survey of US medical school curriculum deans, plus a similar survey of residents and fellows at Washington University in St. Louis, and a query of the Association of American Medical Colleges (AAMC) Curriculum

Inventory database for keywords associated with Cannabis Medicine. The article reports:

> *"The majority of deans (66.7%) reported that their graduates were not at all prepared to prescribe medical marijuana, and 25.0% reported that their graduates were not at all prepared to answer questions about medical marijuana. The vast majority of residents and fellows (89.5%) felt not at all prepared to prescribe medical marijuana, while 35.3% felt not at all prepared to answer questions, and 84.9% reported receiving no education in medical school or residency on medical marijuana. Finally, only 9% of medical school curriculums documented in the AAMC Curriculum Inventory database held content on medical marijuana."*[132]

Yet, according to prominent traditional medical doctors who have conducted research into Cannabis Medicine, knowledge of the ECS will override the current medical system of managing and treating disease symptoms after disease has occurred, and instead will create a system of *disease prevention* by manipulating the ECS.[133] Research is already demonstrating tremendous preventative potential with cannabinoid therapies. There is no reason for medical doctors to remain in the dark about this important physiologic system. So, the question remains, why has it apparently been intentionally excluded from the curriculums of medical schools?

One major reason is the ECS was discovered by scientists studying the active compounds in marijuana, a taboo subject that has always been discouraged by the powers that be. Rather than expressing any interest in, or curiosity about, the promising body of research being developed around the medical promise of cannabinoids, the federal government has blindly held firm to its classification of cannabis as a Schedule 1 Controlled Substance, which was inaccurate in the first place, but politically motivated.

Dedicated researchers who decided they care enough about how Cannabis Medicine works to buck the status quo uncovered the first cannabinoid receptors in 1988. Then in 1991, scientists realized human bodies naturally generate chemical compounds remarkably similar to the ones in cannabis plants, and the plant-generated compounds mimic the physiologic activities of these naturally occurring chemical compounds in human bodies.

Scientists began to realize these chemical compounds make up a complex communication network throughout the entire body, with a particularly strong presence in the brain, central nervous system, and immune system. This communication network functions as a biological balancing mechanism to ensure homeostasis throughout the body. The system, the ECS, has been proven to affect a broad range of health-related issues as diverse as chronic pain, tumor growth, metabolic diseases, mood disorders, epilepsy, and many more. Cannabinoids, whether generated by human bodies or by cannabis plants, ease multiple symptoms produced by a vast array of diseases, disorders, and conditions.

Despite these incredible discoveries, though, cannabis has remained a controlled substance, classified by the US federal government as Schedule 1, a category for chemical compounds that have no accepted medical use. The key word here is "accepted," not proven, or even potential. The American Medical Association initially opposed prohibiting its use, according to *Scientific American*, which also reported that by 1944 the La Guardia Committee Report from the New York Academy of Medicine questioned making cannabis illegal.[134] And yet, the powerful powers that be appear to have a vested interested in ignoring this taboo topic rather than pursuing knowledge and understanding of its true medicinal promise.

WHAT, EXACTLY, IS THE ECS?

The ECS is a control system involving tissue receptor proteins, cellular communication and control, molecular anatomy, and scavenging oxygen free radicals. Additionally, the ECS is a molecular system whose role is to regulate and balance numerous body systems and bodily processes, including cellular communication and immune response.

Unlike other systems in the human body, the ECS is not made up of an independent structure. Rather, the ECS is composed of receptors located on every cell throughout the entire body. These receptors are activated by a set of specific ligands (molecules that bind to receptors), collectively known as endogenous cannabinoids, or endocannabinoids, which are cannabinoids produced within and by the human body. Endocannabinoids regulate a wide range of physiological processes; they are key components of cellular membranes that are produced on demand, and they are hydrophobic, meaning they cannot travel very far in the body, so their effects are localized. These qualities make the ECS unique among systems in the human body.

Endocannabinoids interact with receptors in multiple ways by signaling, controlling, and regulating a range of metabolic functions. They are not unique to humans, but are found in all animal species. An ECS is present and functioning in both vertebrate and invertebrate animals, indicating it originated with or before the last common ancestor of these two major groups, which split apart over 600 million years ago. Reports of using cannabis for medicinal purposes have been traced back as far as 2700 BCE, and even at that time they were apparently being used for their neuroprotective effects.

The ECS involves three core components:

- endocannabinoids
- receptors
- enzymes

THE ENDOCANNABINOID SYSTEM

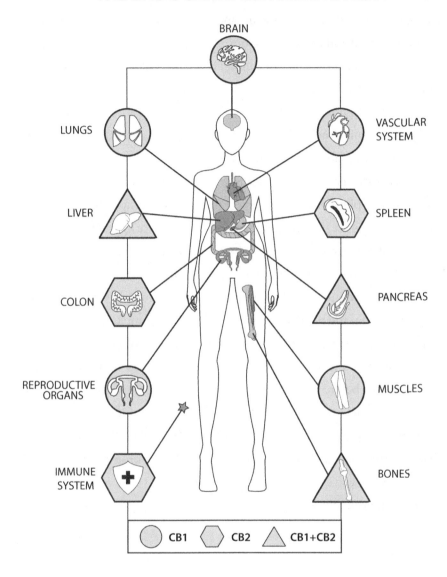

ENDOCANNABINOIDS

Endocannabinoids are chemical compounds produced by the human body that work within the ECS. They are produced in the synapse of neurons (nerve cells) in the central nervous system (CNS), and released in response to various biological signals providing precise, essential information about the state of certain biological processes. Endocannabinoids are then produced and released according to the need for regulating those processes.

There are two major endocannabinoids:

- Anandamide
- 2-AG

These endocannabinoids are produced in the body from fat-like molecules in cell membranes. They bind directly to and activate cannabinoid receptors. Endocannabinoids are synthesized on-demand, meaning they are produced and used exactly when and where they're needed, rather than being stored for later use, like many other biological molecules.

ENDOCANNABINOID RECEPTORS

An important class of cell membrane receptors located throughout the body, endocannabinoid receptors bind directly to endocannabinoids in order to signal that something has gotten out of balance and needs to be corrected. Receptors are like locks and the ligand compounds that bind to them are like the keys in a lock & key system. Endocannabinoids can bind to either of two receptors which sit on the surface of cells and monitor conditions outside the cell. They transmit information about changing conditions outside the cell to the inside of the cell, initiating appropriate cellular responses.

In humans and other mammals, the ECS is made up of two main cannabinoid receptors, known as CB1 and CB2, in addition to a number of other secondary receptors that influence the actions of the main receptors:

CB1 receptors:

- Are one of the most prevalent receptors in the brain,
- Are found in dense concentrations throughout the brain, central nervous system, and peripheral nervous system,
- Are found in the pituitary, adrenal, and thyroid glands, in fat, muscle,

and liver cells, and in the digestive tract, lungs, and kidneys,

- Are found in immune cells, but in lower concentration than the CB2 receptors,
- Interact with various cannabinoids, but not all cannabinoids bind perfectly to the CB1 receptors,
- Are crucial for regulating homeostasis in body temperature, fluid balance, appetite and food intake, blood sugar levels, ion concentration, inflammation, and many other related functions.

CB2 receptors:
- Are generally found in the peripheral nervous system, the spleen, thymus gland, tonsils, gastrointestinal system, and certain immune cells,
- Are present in the brain and central nervous system, but at much lower density than CB1 receptors,
- Appear to primarily regulate immunological responses such as inflammation, cell migration, and programmed cell death,
- Play a crucial role in the regulation of bone mass, bone density, and overall bone health,
- Interact with various ligands in different ways and to differing extents.

These are not the only cannabinoid receptors, but they are the most prevalent. They were the first ones identified, and they are the most-studied, so they are the best-understood. Most cannabinoids, whether generated by human bodies or by cannabis plants, can bind to both CB1 & CB2 receptors. However, CBD doesn't directly trigger either receptor. Instead, it modifies the receptors' ability to bind to other cannabinoids.

Receptors are proteins located on the surface of cells that interact with substances outside the cell to produce a response inside the cell. The substances that interact with the receptors are known as ligands, and they generally interact with the receptors in one of three ways:

1. **Agonist:** If a ligand binds to a receptor and produces an effect, it is an agonist.

2. **Antagonist:** If a ligand binds to a receptor and produces no effect, it is an antagonist.
   - These substances can be useful because they block the receptor from being utilized by an agonist.

3. **Inverse Agonist:** If a ligand binds to a receptor and produces the opposite effect from that of an agonist, it is known as an inverse agonist.
   - Inverse agonists can also be blocked by antagonists.

There is also a fourth important way ligands interact with receptors -- as Allosteric Modulators, which bind to different parts of a receptor and modulate the action of an agonists in subtle ways. Allosteric modulators are a group of substances that bind to receptors to change how they respond to stimulus:

- A positive allosteric modulator increases the biological activity of an agonist.
- A negative allosteric modulator decreases the biological activity of an agonist.

METABOLIC ENZYMES

Metabolic enzymes synthesize and break down the endocannabinoids after they've been used. The two most important enzymes in the ECS are:

- FAAH, which breaks down anandamide,
- MAGL, which breaks down 2-AG.

These enzymes ensure endocannabinoids are used when and where they're needed, but only as long as necessary. This quality distinguishes endocannabinoids from other molecular signals in the body.

Neurotransmitters are molecules that transmit messages between brain cells, or neurons, and from neurons through the rest of the body. Similar to the way serotonin and dopamine are chemical messengers, or neurotransmitters, for the nervous system, endocannabinoids are neurotransmitters for the ECS. Brain cells communicate with each other and with the cells from other parts of the body by sending chemical messages that help coordinate and regulate bodily activities. Neurotransmitters, the messenger chemicals, are typically released from the presynaptic cell, then travel across a small gap, the synapse, and attach to specific receptors located on a nearby neuron, the postsynaptic cell. This process stimulates the receiving neuron into action and initiates a set of events that allow the message to be passed along.

Interestingly, the ECS works backward. When the postsynaptic neuron is activated, cannabinoids are produced from lipid precursors that already exist within the neuron. They are released from the postsynaptic cell and travel backward to the presynaptic neuron, where they attach to cannabinoid receptors. Since cannabinoids act on presynaptic cells, they influence what happens next. By traveling backward, the molecular message is actually received by the presynaptic neuron, so the effect is to increase the number of cannabinoid receptors located on the postsynaptic neuron. Endocannabinoids are produced as needed, depending on the desired activity level, and then released from the postsynaptic neurons, travel backward across the synapse, activate the presynaptic cannabinoid receptors, and regulate the presynaptic function. This way, binding with the neurotransmitters being released from the presynaptic neuron will cause another increase of neurotransmission until a strong communication is formed. Endocannabinoids control the activity level for presynaptic neurons, affecting the amount of neurotransmitter that is released, which in turn affects how cellular messages are communicated and processed.

Most cannabinoids can bind with both CB1 and CB2 receptors, but CBD doesn't directly act on either. Rather, it works by changing the receptors' ability to bind with other cannabinoids, influencing the way the ECS works. CBD also inhibits the enzymes that prevent other cannabinoids from accomplishing their maximum effect, preventing them from zooming into overdrive.

HOMEOSTASIS

The tendency of a system, especially the physiological system of higher animals, to maintain internal stability, owing to the coordinated response of its parts to any situation or stimulus that would tend to disturb its normal condition or function. —Dictionary.com

Understanding the biological concept of homeostasis is critically important for understanding the ECS. Homeostasis is a state of stability, equilibrium, and balance. In human bodies, homeostasis is accomplished through essential systems working to stabilize the internal environment, allowing the body to function smoothly and efficiently. As the environment fluctuates, biological responses ebb and flow accordingly. When necessary, chemical messengers are released into the bloodstream, triggering mechanisms that work to maintain the extremely delicate internal balance.

Human bodies don't function at their best if the internal temperature is too hot or too cold, blood pressure or blood sugar levels are too high or too low, etc. Conditions need to be just right for cells to perform optimally, so precise systems work continuously to ease them back into balance when they shift out. Because of its extensive influence over homeostasis, the ECS regulates the biochemistry involved with processes that adjust for changes in the internal environment. Strategies to maintain homeostasis are ongoing throughout every system of the body, and luckily, if you experience a disruption in one function, say an upset stomach or a tension headache, the other bodily functions all generally manage to continue performing their specific tasks without missing a beat. These complex functions, and many others, play unique roles to help keep the body performing at ideal efficiency. Automatic control systems throughout the body are constantly making precise adjustments to maintain optimal vital conditions like temperature, oxygen levels, and hydration.

The ECS is the primary homeostatic regulatory system of the body. It can adjust specific distinct processes when needed without having any effect on others. Total homeostasis of the entire body is a reflection of the combined relative homeostasis of each variable in the body. However, if any system reaches a point that it can no longer achieve or maintain homeostasis, the imbalance could ultimately devolve into illness, disease, or other health issues. Few of us bother to think about the intricate miracles involved with things like digestion and metabolism, but they are nothing short of magical.

Understanding how the ECS works to maintain homeostasis is key to understanding how cannabinoid medicine could help ease various medical conditions. For example, inflammation is the body's natural protective response to an infection or physical damage, and it plays an important role in the healing process. An area becomes inflamed when fluid and immune cells migrate to the damaged tissues in order to quash infection and attack foreign invaders, like a splinter or a bee stinger, or irritants like viruses and bacteria. Healthy inflammation is limited to the damaged location, and doesn't linger any longer than needed.

But unhealthy inflammation leads to systemic imbalances in the body and promotes the negative effects of oxidative stress. Extended disruptions of homeostasis can cause chronic inflammation, which ultimately leads to autoimmune diseases where the immune response doesn't shut off, but instead kicks into overdrive and attacks healthy cells. The ECS is instrumental in managing the processes that resolve inflammation and regulate the immune response, returning the affected systems to homeostasis.

Inflammation in the central nervous system plays a significant role in the development of numerous neurodegenerative diseases, including

Alzheimer's and Parkinson's, as well as multiple sclerosis, Lupus, and others. Many diseases that humans are genetically predisposed to are inflammation-related. When cannabinoids bind to the receptors on neurons, messages are sent to the nucleus of each cell and appropriate action is then taken so the cells return to homeostasis. The main forces of balance in the central nervous system are grouped into two categories:

- Relaxation/inhibition,
- Excitation.

When the neurons of the central nervous system become relaxed/inhibited, the person will often experience difficulty with mobility and/or drowsiness. On the other hand, when elements of the central nervous system become overly excited, conditions like anxiety, migraines, or insomnia can be triggered.

Cannabinoids, whether generated by human bodies or by cannabis plants, attach to receptors throughout the body and activate certain chemical molecules known as neurotransmitters to transport messages. For example, CBD up-regulates the immune genes that create anti-inflammatory biochemicals that reduce inflammation in the central nervous system. CBD also up-regulates the GABA-system that produces feelings of calm and relaxation. On the other hand, CBD down-regulates the genes that cause inflammation in the immune system and the glutamate system, which provoke over-excitement.

The ECS is a lipid signaling system critically involved in the regulation of energy balance. Metabolism relies on a balance between anabolism and catabolism, processes that work to help organize molecules by releasing and capturing energy to keep the body functioning smoothly. Anabolism centers around growth, building, and organizing molecules; small, simple molecules are built up into larger, more complex ones. Increases in muscle mass are a good example of anabolic processes. On the other hand, catabolism breaks down molecules to be used as energy; large, complex molecules are broken down into smaller, simple ones. Breaking down the fat in adipose tissue to fatty acids is an example of catabolism. The ECS controls the entire balancing process.[135]

Furthermore, the ECS controls several metabolic functions by acting on tissues in the gastrointestinal tract, skeletal muscles, and the pancreas, which produces insulin. To ensure the body is functioning properly, millions of pancreatic cells produce insulin to maintain stable blood sugar levels. If energy intake becomes unbalanced, the ECS becomes dysregulated and hyperactive in numerous organs that work to maintain energy balance. Homeostatic imbalance can lead to several cardio-metabolic risk factors for obesity and type 2 diabetes. Dysregulation of the ECS is a major factor in building up of excess visceral fat and reducing the flow of hormones released from adipose tissue.[136] CBD lowers this kind of dysregulation, and therefore limits the effects of, and the amount of time for, the resulting imbalance to wreak havoc.

CBD also interacts with the ECS indirectly through multiple targets beyond regular receptors. For example, CBD delays re-uptake of natural neurotransmitters like FAAH, the enzyme that degrades anandamide. CBD affects binding action of G-coupled protein receptors involved in a wide range of biological and neurological processes, including addiction, appetite, sleep, and pain perception.[137] At high concentrations, CBD directly activates 5-HT1A serotonin receptors, causing an anti-anxiety effect.[138]

Additionally, CBD interacts directly with certain ion channels to cause beneficial effects. For example, it binds to TRPV1 receptors, which also function as ion channels and are known to decrease pain perception, inflammation, and body temperature. CBD works as an antagonist that blocks, or deactivates, other G protein-coupled receptors, known as GPR55, that support osteoclast cell function, which facilitates bone reabsorption. Overactive GPR55 receptor signaling is associated with osteoporosis, so blocking these receptors helps decrease the negative effects of osteoporosis.[139]

CBD slows cancer cell proliferation, providing anti-cancer effects by activating peroxisome proliferator activated receptors (PPARs), a group of nuclear receptor proteins that regulate gene expression. Activating a receptor known as PPAR-gamma causes tumors in lung cancer cell lines to deteriorate. CBD also reduces brain cancer and breast cancer cell proliferation and metastasis by inhibiting the expression of the ID-1 gene, which plays a role in several kinds of aggressive cancers.[140]

Additionally, CBD promotes PPAR-alpha activity by inhibiting FAAH, the metabolic enzyme that breaks down several endogenous fatty acid compounds, including anandamide. CBD modulates receptors on the surface of nuclei, regulating gene expression and mitochondrial activity. CBD functions as a PPAR-gamma agonist, degrading a key molecule linked to the development of Alzheimer's disease. PPAR receptors also regulate genes that are involved in energy homeostasis, lipid uptake, insulin sensitivity, and other metabolic functions, so it has multiple positive effects.[141] CBD works with the ECS in numerous other ways to help maintain, or regain, homeostasis in every physiologic system, and ultimately total homeostasis of human bodies.

When we imagine how the impressive medical research conducted over the past 30 years could likely have accomplished so much more if it had included the ECS, we feel a combination of exasperation that it didn't, coupled with hope for future advancements when the ECS is acknowledged in a way that will allow medical research to become more thorough and complete. Until that time, at least the wheels are beginning to roll, as demonstrated by the examples listed above.

CLINICAL ENDOCANNABINOID DEFICIENCY SYNDROME

Clinical Endocannabinoid Deficiency (CED) is a theory proposing certain health conditions and their symptoms develop when the body's ECS is not functioning properly. CED was originally based on the concept that certain brain disorders develop because of neurotransmitter deficiencies, like Parkinson's disease resulting from dopamine deficiency. A similar idea, that a deficiency in the ECS could trigger the development of certain disorders, is the main premise of CED. The theory suggests that, at least in some cases, the ECS may not be working correctly because either the body isn't producing enough endocannabinoids or adequate receptors for the ECS to function properly. Homeostasis becomes compromised, and when the body is out-of-balance, compromised conditions can lead to the development of diseases.

The theory of CED was originally proposed in 2004 by Dr. Ethan Russo, a renowned cannabinoid researcher who is a board-certified neurologist and psychopharmacology researcher. Dr. Russo is Past-President of the International Cannabinoid Research Society, and former Chairman of the International Association for Cannabinoid Medicines. Clearly, he is truly an expert in the field. In 2004, Dr. Russo published a study in the journal *Neuro Endocrinology Letters,* where he suggested that deficient cannabinoid levels might be the reason why some health conditions develop.[142] He suggested that deficiencies of this sort could explain why supplementing with plant cannabinoids was proving to be effective for easing the symptoms of certain conditions. His initial research focused on migraine, fibromyalgia, and irritable bowel syndrome, but over time, with continued research, CED has been linked to many other disorders.

Dr. Russo proposed that increasing the ECS activity level with cannabinoid agonists might ease many health problems. Most experts agree that correcting CED could probably be approached with one of three strategies:

1. Increase cannabinoids, either by stimulating the body's production of endocannabinoids, enhancing with plant-derived cannabinoids, or both.

2. Decrease the breakdown of endocannabinoids.

3. Increase/decrease receptor density and/or function as needed.

Although using cannabis plants, either hemp or marijuana, to increase cannabinoid levels is one obvious strategy for jump-starting the ECS, others have emerged.

Alongside Dr. Russo, many other scientists have contributed to the body of research surrounding CED, and a variety of theories have been suggested as possible strategies for manipulating the ECS. One thing that has become clear is that food intake can definitely affect endocannabinoid levels. One incredibly easy strategy is to boost omega-3 fatty acid intake, because omega-3s are the building blocks for forming CB1 receptors. Hemp seeds are one of the most abundant and healthy sources of omega-3 fatty acids, plus other seeds and legumes are high in omega-3 and omega-6 fatty acids; fish oil supplements are also a good option. A specific terpene, caryophyllene, found in a variety of herbs and spices like cloves, rosemary, basil, oregano, and black pepper, stimulates endocannabinoid receptors by binding to them. Another dietary influence on the ECS is high quality dark chocolate, which boosts anandamide levels, plus it calms the brain and increases neural activity. Carrots contain a compound called falcarinol that interacts with both CB1 and CB2 receptors and causes a reaction at the CB1 receptors. Simply drinking regular dairy milk can boost the ECS, as it contains 2-AG.

Another strategy suggests addressing a low-functioning ECS with exercise. In addition to all the other benefits from exercise, it also increases anandamide and boosts CB1 receptors in the brain, which helps reduce pain perception.[143] Other strategies include managing stress and limiting alcohol consumption, because high levels of cortisol, the stress hormone, impede CB1 receptor function, and both stress and heavy alcohol indulgence slow the growth of new endocannabinoid receptors.

The theory of CED is based on scientific studies, but so far, none of the research offers guidance on how cannabinoids, including CBD, would best be used to adjust an under-performing ECS. CBD is safe and non-intoxicating, so it is used by people seeking relief from conditions that are theoretically caused by CED, like migraine, fibromyalgia, and IBS. The idea that anandamide is crucial for reducing CED-based diseases leads to the possibility of using CBD to inhibit FAAH to compromise the break-down of anandamide. Additionally, CBD directly affects serotonin receptors in the brain by binding and activating the 5-HT1A receptors, which is one of the ways CBD works to ease anxiety. CBD and other cannabinoids offer tremendous potential for changing the course of CED-based diseases.

THE CUTANEOUS ECS

Skin has its own ECS that produces both anandamide and 2-AG, which are synthesized by numerous cell types throughout the epidermis, hair follicles, and sebaceous glands. The primary function of the skin's ECS is basically the same as that of the ECS throughout the rest of the body: maintaining homeostasis. The skin's ECS is applicable to numerous skin cell functions, including proliferation, survival, and differentiation, which are essential elements in the delicate balance of skin homeostasis. The skin's ECS influences a wide variety of biological processes like cell growth, proliferation, and differentiation, plus hormone production, and mediation of skin cells like hair follicles and sebaceous glands.

The primary physiological function of the skin's ECS is to manage cell growth, maturation, survival, and skin cell death. Classic CB1 and CB2 receptors exist in almost all types of skin cells. CB1 receptors are common in human hair follicles, and CB2 receptors are typical on sebaceous glands. Endocannabinoid signaling is associated with conditions like dermatitis, wound healing, melanoma, and many others. Disturbances of the delicate homeostatic balance of the skin's ECS can produce various skin conditions, including:

- Acne,

- Seborrhea, or excessive discharge of sebum from sebaceous glands,

- Allergic dermatitis,

- Itchiness,

- Hair growth disorders,

- Systemic sclerosis, an autoimmune disorder that changes the texture and appearance of skin.[144]

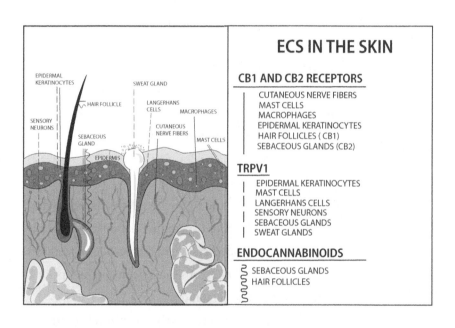

Skin's natural fats, called lipids, play an important role in protecting skin from damage and in retaining moisture. Lipids are also involved with skin's natural repair processes. Both anandamide and 2AG enhance cellular responses from essential genes involved with lipid synthesis. Because the skin's ECS plays such an integral role in skin health, researchers are interested in exploring how cannabinoids, including CBD, could manage common skin problems including:

Psoriasis, a condition caused by skin cells multiplying 10 times faster than normal, resulting in bumpy red patches covered with white scales. Because the ECS inhibits cell growth and encourages cell death, cannabinoid agonists could help with managing psoriasis.

Acne, which is stimulated by increased sebum, the oily substance created by sebaceous glands that helps keep skin and hair moisturized. Activating CB2 receptors helps slow sebum production. Stabilizing the skin's ECS helps balance sebum production.

Dermatitis or inflammation of the skin, which usually presents as red, dry, itchy skin, but can lead to more serious issues like painful cracked skin, blisters that secrete fluid, and crusty, scaly skin. Balancing the ECS helps manage skin inflammation.[145]

CLOSING THOUGHTS

The ECS is a complicated system, and politics have created some huge obstacles to the processes of learning about and understanding the intricate workings of this amazing system. No other system in human bodies works the way the ECS does, and many people believe it should be the highest priority for future medical professionals to understand.

The fact that it was only discovered relatively recently, coupled with the fact that it has been systematically withheld from science and medical education, do not mean it is not real. The ECS is not a proposed theory, it is very real, and it has the potential to guide the medical establishment into new frontiers of patient care. Cannabinoids, whether generated by human bodies or by cannabis plants, have been proven to ease multiple symptoms associated with a vast array of diseases, disorders, and conditions. Ideas about how to work with this system to help people living with chronic health conditions are vast and varied.

The American Medical Association has been against limiting cannabinoids for therapeutic uses. We salute those doctors who have taken the initiative to become informed about the ECS, and suggest to other medical professionals that learning about the ECS and becoming knowledgeable about making safe and appropriate recommendations for cannabinoid therapies, including CBD, is not only appropriate, it is truly imperative considering the efficacy and popularity of Cannabis Medicine.

BOLD EXPLORERS
BLAZING THE TRAIL

MY NAME IS ANDRA, and I can say with great surprise and excitement that CBD has changed my life in every good way possible. I want to share my success story because I want to give you hope that there are effective alternatives to treating disorders, diseases, and symptoms.

I have lived with chronic illnesses most of my life. I have a background in holistic healing and have also been in the cannabis industry for fifteen years plus, though it literally took me years to try and find a CBD product that actually worked for me. I have finally found an astoundingly effective complementary medicine that I had always searched for yet had decided didn't exist. I am here to tell you it is real. It is natural. It works.

From a young age I can remember often having excruciating knee pain. At one point my mother took me to a specialist who said I should have had knee surgery as an infant and that when I was 30, I would have the back of a 60-year-old. Well, that wasn't very encouraging for a young child to hear. Like most children I played outdoor games and athletic sports, but I was the slowest and I always had pain. I gave it my best, but I suffered.

In high school it worsened and my attention span decreased, as it is hard to focus when in severe pain. At the age of sixteen I had arthroscopic surgery on each knee, a month apart from each other. After that, for recovery I did physical therapy by swimming laps every day. By this time, I was taking anti-inflammatories and muscle relaxers on a regular basis. I did not like the way they made me feel, but I liked having less pain. There were more sleepless nights than restful ones at times. I have always loved being active, but I always pay for it with the resulting pain. I have also endured great fatigue since childhood. That would be my other dominant symptom. These two things, pain and fatigue, made life challenging and

I just wanted to be a regular kid that felt great and had energy to play.

See, I grew up with a father who was a pharmacist for fifty-five years, and for twenty-five of those years he was the chief pharmacist at our local hospital. That being said, I was raised with western medicine as a treatment for any symptoms or disease. I feel fortunate to have some understanding of western medicine and what it offers us. Traditional medicine has its place, as it allows for and gives diagnostics, pharmaceutical medicines, and surgery. Western medicine is also quite heroic as it saves many lives. Needless to say, I have a healthy respect for traditional medicine and I am grateful we live in these times of advanced technology. My father did me a great service by giving me information and knowledge, and leading me to my passion for medicine and the healing path.

At the age of twenty-one I moved to Santa Fe, New Mexico to attend massage therapy school. Studying alternative therapies challenged my beliefs about health and healing which changed the course of my life forever. As I began my journey into natural health, I discovered a plethora of modalities, techniques, teachings, and systems. All I knew was that I wanted to feel better. I was there to heal myself then give back by assisting others in their own healing process. While in school, I was introduced to a whole new world. I took these tools with me and continued to use them.

I carried these alternative practices into motherhood and the way I parent. They became a way of life. I still struggled with pain and fatigue as my main symptoms. Often, I feel body pain completely all over and throughout me. Although mothering has been my greatest joy, I remember the immense effort it took to perform all the tasks necessary to raise three children who were safe, healthy, and happy while keeping our household going. I remember after having children, my overall body pain and fatigue worsened.

During my childbearing and childrearing years I was adamantly holistic. I had each of my children naturally with no medication or pain prevention methods. I was very clear, determined, and set on specific experiences that I wanted for my family, beginning from birth.

Fast forward into my early 30s. After much inspiration and self-will, I found working out to become my tonic and passion. I lifted weights, did cardio, yoga, walked, hiked, rock climbed outdoors and indoors. I was very focused on being active and maybe a little obsessed, as I did activities six or seven days a week. It kept me sane and I was not in as much pain. I had more energy, which was a great motivator. Eventually, though, I hit a very large brick wall. My body was spent and the universe had other plans for me. After a series of health crises occurred, that was the end of my athletic stint.

Not long after that, I began studying naturopathic medicine. I loved my classes and it just felt like an extension of the work I had begun in massage therapy school. It was a way of life and became even more so. While the kids were at school, my days were spent studying and resting on the couch. My pain and fatigue were at their worst. By this time, I had tried what I thought was every alternative therapy under the sun. You name it, I had tried it, to no avail. Nothing, no modalities, therapies, or treatments helped me with the pain and fatigue. I was more than discouraged, I was distraught and resigned. I was not functioning and I was suffering.

I finally decided to seek western medical attention, and was diagnosed with Fibromyalgia and Chronic Fatigue Syndrome. I was shocked, yet it finally made sense and I had my long-awaited answer. I was relieved to have a diagnosis and know I wasn't crazy or lazy. It was not the answer I wanted, but at least it gave me more to work with.

Still in immense pain, my doctor at the time offered me pain medication. I took it once a day. That was the most compassionate thing anyone could have done for me then. I believe everything has its time and place. It was time for relief, and at that point I was desperate and willing to try anything, even if it meant using traditional pharmaceutical medicines again.

I was relieved and very grateful that the pain medicine did take the edge off, although the pain never fully subsided. I just got really good at putting it on the back burner and living with it and the fatigue like I had been doing my whole life.

As you may guess, over time I needed more and more medication to control my pain. My body developed a dependency on it, and going without it was no longer an option. There were many times my dose had to increase to control the symptoms or a new medication was required and introduced. There were also times I decided to cut down or wean myself off medication, with the doctor's supervision of course. Still, at this point I had accepted that I would be on medication to control the pain for the rest of my life. That was a very defeating and sobering realization to know I would have to rely on these meds to function at all from there on out.

During this period, my doctor asked if I had ever tried cannabis and suggested I use it for symptomatic relief from the fibromyalgia. So, I tried it, and I felt like it helped me differently than the pharmaceutical medication. I began using cannabis regularly and medicated several times a day with positive effects. Eventually, I became a medical grower myself so I could provide my own organic product, knowing exactly what went into the flower I was using as medicine.

As the years went by and the industry grew and marijuana was legalized in my state, I've had the opportunity to try many cannabis products, including CBD. I was never impressed or had any experiences with relief from those CBD products, though. It was always disappointing so I dismissed CBD as something that would not work for me. At the time I did not understand Cannabis Medicine. Little did I know that someday I would find the right CBD product for me. Well, I did, and my life has changed forever.

In August of 2021 I was introduced to a CBD tincture that had added CBG, CBN and CBC. I started on a very low dose to see how my body would do. Honestly, I noticed very little on the lower dose. I felt calmer, yet I was still having fibromyalgia pain. I increased my dose and on day five I awoke feeling quite different. I sat up and realized I had no pain. Not only that, but I felt great and had more energy than I knew what to do with in that moment. I felt no pain! I asked myself, "Is this how other people feel? Wow!" At that point I was literally in shock and quite giddy with disbelief. Maybe I got the right amount of sleep. Maybe yesterday didn't wear me out. Maybe it was one of those rare good day, I thought. As the day went on, and then the next several days, I continued with my new regimen of CBD, in no fibromyalgia pain, and still completely shocked and happily surprised.

I also found that my ADHD was quieting down. I began focusing better. I felt calmer and not as anxious. I stayed on a moderate dose, adjusting when necessary. Now I have found a maintenance dose that is right for me. If I don't take it, my body always reminds me when I need it, so I've learned to listen. When I begin to notice fibromyalgia pain creeping in, I immediately take a dose. Soon after, I always feel relief again.

I know CBD isn't a cure-all for everyone and everything. I can honestly say, though, that it helps me manage at a higher level of functioning. It has increased my quality of life. Because of the CBD, I also have more quantity of life. I get to do more activities and be more comfortable at the same time. CBD has far surpassed any expectations I've ever had about finding a natural way to heal and promote a sense of overall well-being. I could not be more thrilled and excited with the results I am having and I will continue to use CBD as part of my life and my healing path.

Chapter

5

CANNABIS PLANT MEDICINE: STORY AND SCIENCE, A PRESCRIPTION FOR HEALTH

BY DR. SHARON MONTES, M.D.

MY CAREER AS A HOLISTIC DOCTOR who uses plant medicine was influenced by being the daughter of an artist mother and scientist father who were united by their love of nature. Large gardens, nature walks, and learning about edible and medicinal wild plants were deeply woven into my childhood. I grew up understanding plants are inherent partners in creating and sustaining health, both as food and as medicine. I always considered myself lucky to have been born into a family that used nutrition, meditation, prayer, and plant medicine blended with science.

We always had a large garden brimming with fruits and vegetables, plus an assortment of herbs that went far beyond the standard mint and basil. I knew early on that echinacea, also known as cone flower, is effective at treating a variety of ailments, including wounds, burns, toothaches, sore throat, and upset stomach, though it's most often used to treat or prevent common colds. In my family, we gathered "weeds" that were used for food and medicine. Later, in medical school, I realized that offering patients herbal remedies for viral infections was safer and more effective than the medicines I learned about in pharmacology class.

For thousands of years, humans have been developing mutually beneficial relationships with other species, from dogs and cats to plants and bacteria. These relationships are examples of mutualistic coevolution, which happens when multiple species have a positive effect on each other's progress over time, allowing different life forms to evolve together and flourish. Humanity has developed an "evolutionary garden," a collection of plants and fungi that people have been cultivating since prehistory and have transported around the world because they are useful for health and survival. One of the plants in the evolutionary garden, cannabis, has been evolving all across this planet for tens of millions of years, originating from its hardy ancestors in central Asia.

Early cannabis traces back to when the Himalayas were forming. Sixty million years ago, those mountains were formed by the Indian subcontinent crashing into the Asian plate. All life in the region had to either adapt or die. Plants became hardy in order to survive, creating a unique opportunity for cannabis' ancestral plant, which appeared 40 to 50 million years ago, to become extremely versatile. Over the millions of years since, cannabis has been able to survive in a variety of climates, and to truly thrive in many of them.

In response to the harsh environment near the Himalayas, cannabis began to produce a wide range of chemicals the human body is particularly well suited to process. The cannabis plant has over 500 chemicals, like cannabinoids and terpenes, that are known to have beneficial health effects. Chemically, plant cannabinoids work to create and maintain balance at the cellular level by working with the ECS. It is a bit confusing, but the human system is named for chemicals found in plants. The endocannabinoid system relies on cannabinoid receptors found in human brains and throughout the entire human body.

Humans' relationship with cannabis can be traced back through thousands of years of documentation about the uses of this plant, plus oral histories that reach back even farther. However, despite my deeply ingrained belief that plants have essential healing qualities, I found myself unable to get excited about the idea of cannabis as medicine in the early years of legalization.

There were not many guidelines for using Cannabis Medicine, so many people referred to the cannabis industry as the "Wild, Wild West," a term that rings deeply in the hearts of many Coloradoans. We've always considered ourselves pioneers of one sort or another, and Colorado has been a pioneer in the arena of legalization for marijuana, for both medical and recreational use. One of the first states to legalize medical marijuana back in 2000, and since then, Colorado was one of only two states blazing the trail for legal adult recreational marijuana in 2014. Though I absolutely share a pioneering spirit with many fellow Coloradoans, I wasn't particularly excited or enthusiastic about working with cannabis as a health care provider. Knowing that it had been illegal for years, I wasn't so quick to see it as the cure-all that many people seemed to think it was. I was skeptical. As a doctor, I had my doubts about one plant with a shady history somehow being able to help so many people with such a wide array of issues.

Furthermore, I had been working in urgent care and had seen several young men who came to me complaining of back pain, who also indicated they got relief from smoking marijuana. At that time, I wasn't familiar with any of the science about the endocannabinoid system, so again, I was skeptical and frankly, judgmental. My cynical mind thought they were looking for a pass to justify getting stoned. On the other hand, my logical mind somehow also knew that smoking marijuana was a hundred times safer than using opioids or self-medicating with alcohol. I wasn't sure about its pain-relieving potential, but I was certain that smoking marijuana would help relax the mind and muscles, so I told myself there was no harm if these young men misinterpreted this as physical pain relief. But make no mistake, they were also sent out of urgent care with recommendations for an anti-inflammatory diet and stretching exercises!

My conversion and commitment to become a Cannabis Medicine advocate and educator occurred over time as a result of three significant life events. First, in 2016, I had a patient in my holistic practice who was living with complex nerve pain from the combination of a genetic condition that makes it difficult for her to metabolize and incorporate fatty acids into her cell membranes, coupled with a diagnosis of Lyme disease. She asked me to review a recommendation she had received for medical marijuana from the manager of a local medical marijuana dispensary.* I agreed to take a look at the recommendation she had, and I was impressed when I recognized it was a masterpiece in plant medicine that made full use of a variety of delivery forms including topicals, edibles, smoke, and concentrate. This plant medicine recommendation successfully blended a range of both long-acting and short-acting forms of plant medicine to reduce physical pain and anxiety, and to improve mood and sleep. While I was intrigued and impressed by her plant medicine prescription, I was busy with my practice and happy to let cannabis recommendations be made by "those people" at the dispensaries. I wasn't ready to integrate cannabis into my clinical practice.

*In the state of Colorado (and other states), doctors don't prescribe medical marijuana. They take a medical history and conduct an examination with the patient to verify the person qualifies for a medical marijuana card, and they can make cannabis recommendations, but they don't prescribe.

Second, in 2017 I sent my 83-year-old mother to obtain a medical marijuana card from a local doctor who performed eligibility exams. She lives with severe arthritis and definitely met our state's eligibility requirement of severe pain. She and I both found it to be a horrible experience. The doctor's business card had a picture of a sailboat on it and the words "World Traveler" underneath the image of the boat. I wondered how that related to medical cannabis assessments, but we proceeded through the process up to the point where we tried to use the online registry system, and it didn't work. We spent several months trying to get my mother access to medical marijuana for her arthritis, but we ultimately gave up. The whole experience left a bad taste in my mouth about medical marijuana. I was not impressed with the provider care or the online state registry system.

While these and other experiences seemed to place the idea of Cannabis Medicine in front of me with some regularity, until 2018 I really wasn't on board. In February of 2018, I met a woman who had dedicated the prior 5 years of her life to working with hemp and CBD. She spoke with me about human cell receptors, legacy strains, global distribution of this plant, how humans had interacted with this plant for thousands of years. Her mixture of passion and science broke through my last layer of resistance. My brain lit up! I had a vision of a HUGE cannabis plant that filled a room. For the first time, I had a sense of the essence and power this plant entailed, and I got a sense of how this plant had helped people, as well as the planet. In my heart, I committed to becoming a Cannabis Medicine Ambassador.

Many people get confused between the words Cannabis, hemp, marijuana and the acronyms THC and CBD. For the purpose of this chapter, I will use hemp/CBD to clarify that we are speaking about low THC whole plant products.

Cannabis is a plant that has hundreds of active medicinal chemicals. Two of those chemicals are abbreviated THC and CBD. If cannabis products, meaning the leaves and flower, have more than .03% or .0003 content of THC, the cannabis product is called marijuana. If the product has less than that magic number, then the cannabis product is called hemp.

Many people call their products CBD to emphasize that it is not marijuana. This creates confusion because it is not clear whether the product is whole plant that contains CBD, or if it is an isolate with only one chemical extract. Science is showing that CBD isolate doesn't work as well and has more side effects than whole-plant hemp products.

In order to become a Cannabis Medicine Ambassador, I started with my farmer ancestor roots. I learned of a medicinal hemp farm in my area, and volunteered to help there. I began working with the plant, the people, and the soil, transplanting clones and listening to the other volunteers as they shared their cannabis stories. I learned from a man whose mother grew the plant to make ends meet and shared the medicine with others who were outside the conventional medical system; and from a blind man whose father taught him how to grow the plant; from others whose parents had taught them to grow this amazing plant, who knew how to cook with it. Some people were volunteering on the farm in exchange for product that they shared with loved ones – old people, young people, veterans, animals. I listened to the farmers, including a young man who had left his home in New Mexico because his aunt was living with the diagnosis of breast cancer and he knew this plant could help her. I listened to the founders of the "Fat Pig Society," an all-volunteer organization focused on providing free Hemp/CBD instead of selling it. I was inspired by their vision and their years of commitment dedicated to a cooperative model of growing organic hemp. I found working in the soil with the plant to be a sensory experience, and I found myself celebrating the presence of aphids, ladybugs, and lace wing larvae -- the "good bugs" that eat the "bad bugs."

One thing I was struck by as I continued listening to this diverse assortment of people with such a wide range of backgrounds was that together, we made up an incredibly strong community. We were all sharing our knowledge and wisdom with each other, learning from each other, envisioning how we could continue to use this information to educate others. Both as a doctor and as the plant-medicine enthusiast I had grown up to be, I had a lot of knowledge about plant chemistry. Others had experience working with the soil, and some were expert growers. Each person in this vital community brought their unique combination of expertise, wisdom, and lived experience together. We were definitely stronger than the sum of our individual contributions. After three months of working with the soil, the plants, and especially the people, my scientist brain became engaged in the process.

Among other things, I interviewed 14 different doctors and learned that 13 of them knew absolutely nothing about Cannabis Medicine or the endocannabinoid system, or that their employers were restricting their ability to attend Medical Education conferences. The only doctor I interviewed who did know a little something about the ECS wouldn't advise or consult patients. Rather, he sent his patients to a local CBD store for education if they had questions. (This was before the December 2018 passage of the Farm Bill. Because all cannabis was considered a Schedule 1 dangerous drug by the DEA, many clinicians were "justified" in their fear of stepping into learning or teaching more.) I learned there was a BIG gap between the Plant and the People and the health Providers. Having spent most of my professional life in academics, this fueled my desire to learn more and be of service in bridging the gaps.

One of the interesting things I learned is that cannabinoids are not unique to cannabis. Chemicals that stimulate the human endocannabinoid system are found in many other plants, including echinacea, turmeric, and kava, to name a few, and they are structurally similar to the cannabinoid CBG, the compound that all phytocannabinoids start out as. The ECS is key to overall health and wellness because it regulates all major biological functions. Human bodies continuously strive to operate within a specific state of balance known as homeostasis, and cannabinoids signal the ECS to regain this important equilibrium throughout the body whenever needed.

I began doing some serious research into this system that I had previously never heard of, and I learned the main receptors in the human endocannabinoid system, known as CB1 and CB2, can be traced all the way back to the time when multicellular organisms were developing communication systems that would stimulate action. I learned that cannabinoid receptors are G protein-coupled receptors activated by endocannabinoids, and that these receptors act as molecular switches inside cells. They transmit signals from a variety of stimuli outside a cell to its interior. The activated neurological circuits are important for protecting the brain and other cells. Physical and psychological trauma can disturb the brain or other cells in the body and alter their functioning. The ECS works to maneuver disrupted cells back into optimum functioning, and when necessary, cannabinoids from plants can help keep the process working the way it's designed to work.

I was shocked this information had not been taught in medical school! The ECS is absolutely science-based, and I quickly realized that despite having to learn about it on my own, outside "the ivory tower," it is very real, and of ultimate importance! Throughout the brain and body, cannabinoids play an important role. Their anti-inflammatory and antioxidant properties help the body function at its best at the cellular level. Once they've fulfilled their purpose, endocannabinoids are broken down by enzymes. These chemical compounds are essential to keep internal functions performing efficiently.

Numerous health issues have been linked to improper ECS function. Variables like genetics, stress, nutrition, medications, pollutants, and aging all affect ECS function. Although these are common issues that everyone deals with, they are ECS disruptors. Any of them, or any combination of them, can affect the core components of the ECS in ways that weaken ECS tone and open the possibility of ECS dysfunction. Some conditions associated with clinical endocannabinoid deficiency include:

- Migraines,
- Fibromyalgia,
- Irritable bowel syndrome.

People with low ECS function are likely to have a lower pain threshold, as well as issues with mood, sleep, and digestion. On the other hand, an overactive ECS is associated with conditions like obesity and diabetes. Many doctors, including me, believe balancing the endocannabinoid tone offers a solution to conditions that are otherwise very difficult to treat. In 2016, Dr. Ethan Russo, a true pioneer in medical cannabis research, wrote:

"The theory of Clinical Endocannabinoid Deficiency (CED) was based on the concept that many brain disorders are associated with neurotransmitter deficiencies: affecting acetylcholine in Alzheimer's disease, dopamine in parkinsonian syndromes, serotonin and norepinephrine in depression, and that a comparable deficiency in endocannabinoid levels might be manifest similarly in certain disorders that display predictable clinical features as sequelae of this deficiency."[146]

Russo goes on to explain:

"The greatest evidence for CED is present for migraine, fibromyalgia, and irritable bowel syndrome (IBS). A strong case can be advanced for unifying pathophysiological trends in the three conditions:

- *All manifest hyper-algesic states that must be clinically diagnosed based on subjective criteria as all lack characteristic tissue pathology or easily accessible objective laboratory findings*
- *All are diagnoses of exclusion that often generate extensive negative diagnostic work-ups*

- *They display elevated incidence of anxiety and depression (in a chicken vs. egg dilemma) and have been labeled psychosomatic in origin or worse, wastebasket diagnoses, at one time or another by skeptical clinicians*
- *Comorbidity is quite clear in the three diagnoses. Primary headaches co-occurred in 97% of 201 fibromyalgia patients, 35.6% of 101 chronic daily headache (transformed migraine) subjects also fit clinical criteria of fibromyalgia, and 31.6% of IBS subjects were also diagnosable with fibromyalgia, while 32% of fibromyalgia patients also fit for IBS*
- *While some patients suffer from only one of these syndromes, lifetime risk to develop another, or all three, is quite common."*[147]

The ECS continues holding tight to many of its secrets, but research into its workings is still very new. We do know, however, that certain medications and activities can directly influence it. For example, preclinical trials have demonstrated that nonsteroidal anti-inflammatory medications (NSAIDs) and small doses of opioids enhance endocannabinoid tone, but chronic doses of certain steroids have the opposite effect.

Additionally, lifestyle choices like exercise and stress management affect the ECS. High-intensity exercise tends to boost ECS tone through increased anandamide levels, while chronic stress tends to decrease it. Also, alternative healing modalities like acupuncture and massage directly affect the ECS[148]

Cannabis products offer another strategy for adjusting endocannabinoid tone. One of the reasons most people are successful taking hemp-derived CBD is that it enhances ECS tone. Hemp-derived CBD helps ease pain by acting on a variety of biological processes in the body, as it is an effective anti-inflammatory, antioxidant, and analgesic. Hemp-derived CBD also reduces anxiety that people living with chronic pain often experience.

Cannabis has been used to help alleviate pain since as far back as 2900 BCE, so its use is definitely not new. Both scientific and anecdotal evidence indicate hemp-derived CBD helps people manage chronic pain in a variety of contexts. For example, neuropathic pain is caused by damage to nerves, so it is common with diseases like multiple sclerosis, injuries like herniated discs, and infections like shingles. A 2017 review that looked at 11 randomized controlled trials with 1,219 patients found that hemp-derived CBD helped with chronic neuropathy pain in humans.[149]

A 2016 study in the *European Journal of Pain* used an animal model to explore whether hemp-derived CBD could help people living with arthritis manage their pain. Researchers applied a topical hemp-derived CBD gel to rats that were living with arthritis for 4 days. They noted a significant drop in inflammation and signs of pain, without any additional side effects. People using hemp-derived CBD for arthritis self-report experiencing relief from their pain.[150]

Another study looked at CBD use for general chronic pain. Researchers compiled the results of multiple systematic reviews covering dozens of trials and studies. Their research concluded there is substantial evidence that CBD is effective for chronic pain in adults. Additionally, a study in the *Journal of Experimental Medicine* found that cannabinoids, including CBD, offer helpful new medicinal options to people living with chronic pain.[151] This research not only suggested that using CBD can reduce pain and inflammation, but it also determined that patients were not likely to build up a tolerance to the CBD, so they would not need to increase their dose over time.

There are experts who believe emotional pain and physical pain should be considered as points on a broad pain continuum rather than as fundamentally different. Although some types of pain are purely physical and others are purely emotional, pain often falls somewhere in between these two extremes or encompasses both together. Psychological pain can be intense, and it can affect many areas of life, much like physical pain does. Additionally, psychological pain can contribute to or intensify physical pain. Psychological pain is one of the symptoms often associated with certain mental health conditions.[152]

The most common of these mental health conditions are anxiety disorders and major depression. Stress is a common trigger for both anxiety and depression, as well as many other mental health conditions. Hemp-derived CBD has been well-studied for stress management and prevention. Hemp-derived CBD helps reduce the symptoms of mood disorders, anxiety, depression, sleep issues, fatigue, immune weaknesses, and general stress levels. In addition, CBD is a defense for the adrenal glands, thyroid, and brain against some of the effects of stress. It is also a factor in the body's cortisol and neurotransmitters production.

Many people attempt to manage anxiety and depression using antidepressants, medications primarily used to treat these mental health conditions. However, antidepressants are also increasingly popular as treatments for certain types of chronic physical pain, even when depression isn't considered a factor. Antidepressants increase neurotransmitters in the spinal cord, effectively reducing pain signals, but they don't work immediately. People usually feel some pain relief from an antidepressant after a week or so, but maximum relief usually takes several weeks. If pain relief isn't attained with the antidepressants alone, other medications with distinct mechanisms of pain relief, like anticonvulsants, are sometimes used in combination with antidepressant medications.

Antidepressants are classified based on their chemical structure and how they work. One of the most effective groups of antidepressants for treating pain is known as the tricyclics. Most people are able to take tricyclic antidepressants, particularly in low doses, with only mild side effects. The doses used effectively for pain are generally lower than the doses needed for depression.

Many different classes of antidepressants have been approved by the FDA, including selective serotonin reuptake inhibitors (SSRIs), serotonin and norepinephrine reuptake inhibitors (SNRIs), tricyclic antidepressants, and others. These medications seem to improve symptoms of depression by increasing certain chemicals in the brain like serotonin, norepinephrine, and dopamine to improve mood. However, though these medications were developed years ago and have been improved over many decades in efforts to optimize their effectiveness and reduce their side effects, their exact mechanism remains unclear.

Hemp-derived CBD is emerging as a promising pharmaceutical agent to help with pain, depression, and anxiety, as well as numerous other conditions. Our understanding of the role of CBD in pain management continues to evolve, and evidence from animal studies has shown that CBD exerts its pain-relieving effects through interactions with and modulation of the endocannabinoid, inflammatory, and nociceptive (pain sensing) systems. Given its promising results in animal models, along with its relative safety, absence of psychoactive properties, and low potential for abuse, CBD is an attractive candidate to relieve pain, depression, and anxiety.

Dr. Russo wrote about three specific medical conditions as examples of health conditions that are difficult to treat with traditional western medicine but respond well to Cannabis Medicine. Unfortunately, very few doctors are knowledgeable about how to use Cannabis Medicine, which is really unfortunate for their patients who are suffering with autoimmune disorders, neurological disorders, and/or mental health disorders (as well as many other health issues) that respond so well to CBD. I understand their hesitance and resistance about wanting to delve into this arena of medicine. After studying so long and so hard in medical school, the simplistic idea that a single plant with a sordid history can present viable treatment options that are otherwise not available seems like it must be a crock. When we couple this with the fact that marijuana remains illegal at the federal level, many doctors are not ready to believe CBD, and Cannabis Medicine in general, offer much more than witchcraft or voodoo. I know, because I've been in that exact position.

As I've learned about the workings of the ECS and how it responds to plant cannabinoids like CBD, I've learned new strategies to offer my patients outcomes I couldn't offer them before I gained this knowledge. As I've listened to the wisdom being shared among the members of the strong, vital community I joined through working with the plant and the soil, I realize good medicine is much, much more than the lessons taught in medical school. Like the entourage effect for the chemicals in the cannabis plant working together to complement the benefits of them all, I've learned that people who are committed to learning about the medicinal potential of this plant, and sharing with each other, represent so much more than the sum of the parts. As members of a robust community made up of passionate, caring people, we all have much to share with each other. And the biggest lesson of all is that the future of good medicine will be determined by the trail blazers whose curiosity and personal commitment lead them down the path and through the maze of Cannabis Medicine, and allow themselves to learn about effectively blending traditional western medicine with Cannabis Medicine and other alternative medicinal options.

BOLD EXPLORERS
BLAZING THE TRAIL

I WOULD LIKE TO START OFF by giving a great big THANK YOU to Eric and Catherine for inviting me to share my own story, and a few experiences about how CBD oil has resulted in patients' symptom relief with healing properties unlike any other medicine. I also believe that CBD is valuable as a prospective preventative form of safe, effective, natural medicine.

I graduated with a degree as a certified medical assistant in 1988 and started my career in the healthcare field. I accepted a position at the same office where I performed my clinical and administrative externship with Dr. Carlos Almeida at the Glenn and MaGuire Clinic. Dr. A, as I will refer to him, was a very popular physician and had a private practice in the small town where I was born and raised in central Illinois, where his patients consisted of nearly everyone in town. I had a lot of my "firsts" during this time frame e.g. my first patient that was not a student, my first blood draw on a "real" patient, my first injection to administer, my first healthcare related job, my first time to assist in minor surgery. After a few months. Dr. A announced that he was moving to and joining another local clinic group practice and invited all staff to join him on this new adventure. Every one of his staff, including me, took him up on his offer despite knowing our wages would be significantly decreased; but job security with benefits and the opportunity to continue working with him sealed the deal. I showed up every day and applied all that I had been trained to do and was able to sharpen my clinical and administrative skills. I was offered the opportunity to work as needed up to forty hours every week as a medical records clerk and to float as a medical assistant for the nursing staff. Years later, I was assigned to be Dr. A's hospice RN, which nearly broke my heart. It was both awful and beautiful watching him earn his wings; words cannot express how valuable and miracu-lously rewarding angel work can be.

My career path took a turn in 2001 when I graduated with honors and started my nursing career working locally on skilled care units caring for patients of all ages with a broad spectrum of conditions, disorders, and diseases -- along with administering tons of prescription medications that, right before my eyes (and patients') were leading to chronic kidney and liver failure. I saw first-hand how people's lives and health were being negatively affected by the chemicals in both prescription and over-the-counter medications, as well as from the preservatives and additives in them that the FDA has deemed safe.

Starting in 2009, I worked for five years with Home-Health and Hospice as a case manager and quality control professional employed by my home town hospital.

In the fall of 2015, I received a phone call from my great, dear to my heart friend since middle school, Caprice Sweatt, founder of The Outreach and later owner of CBD stores -- and many other selfless endeavors. Her voice is and was so sincere, inviting me to join in on "spreading the love" and to assist as an RN at clinics, assist with educational events and a few behind the scenes work duties. She introduced me to physicians, and later invited me to work more closely at The Outreach with Eric and Dr. Mauricio Consalter. The vision, mission, and dream to assist others became obvious to me. I consider it all such a huge honor to work with so many amazing like-minded persons in the industry. I am honored and blessed to have the opportunity to incorporate our talents, implementing holistic care to patients, cohorts, colleagues, family, and myself along our wellness journeys. In 2017, after attending an accredited health coaching institute, I became a certified health coach, adding accountability and growth in my knowledge. I now had "more tools in my tool box" to serve our dream of assisting not only ourselves, but also others, with a holistic approach to pain management and wellness, with improved health and quality of life. In July of 2019 I was invited to participate in a CBD seminar held at The CBD Store. There was a small group and I was able to educate them about the hemp history, science in relationship to the endocannabinoid system and how hemp products assist with wellness, dosing suggestions, patient and pet success stories.

Currently, I am unable to perform my nursing and outreach duties due to a motor vehicle accident. Twelve weeks ago, while attempting to avoid a head on collision, I was struck on the drivers' side of my car by a truck entering my lane with very bright headlights, causing me to go off the road while attempting to avoid a hit-and-run accident. This act of "distracted driving" by the other driver resulted in severe injuries to my lower right leg with open compound fractures of both the tibia and fibula, and a crushed heel, along with neck whiplash on my old arthritic bones, exacerbating upper body and right shoulder pain from an old injury. I underwent urgent surgery to apply an external fixator, which led to months of bone healing and decreased mobility due to my non-weight-bearing status. I still face at least two more surgeries and lots of therapy. I have been able to get relief of symptoms including pain, edema, and anxiety with CBD oil. The fact that I had a fixator with rods through my heel and leg bones led us to notice my pain control. During my hospital stay, the nurses and doctors commented on my wound healing process and how, overall, I appeared to have an advanced rate of healing with minimal edema/swelling. This left a door wide open as an opportunity for me to educate and market to healthcare staff about hemp, the amazing natural medicine. I had a captive audience and was marketing The CBD Store and Medical Cannabis Outreach. I love to spread the love!

I shared that I'd been taking CBD oil for my chronic pain in the right shoulder and left knee prior to the accident. I also experienced improved anxiety symptoms and an increased ability to feel balanced, grounded, and focused. The metabolism of each body is unique to every individuals' make up. Throughout my research and self-healing journey over the past 5 years, I have observed that our metabolic rates and overall health are affected by things like prescription medication intake, amount of exercise, food and fluid intake, constant stress, and starving ECSs. Having said that, I have experienced symptom relief related to the anti- inflammatory effects along with balancing effects on nerve receptors; and on a cellular level by feeding my starving ECS with my CBD oil daily dose intake.

This current healing path on my journey involves a holistic approach of positive reframing on a whole new level. In the past, I have experimented by halting my CBD intake for a duration of two to four weeks; my symptoms generally resume within four days. My family and friends have been wonderful, loving, and attentive in assisting with my daily recovery and overall needs while I heal and experience the many layers of transition of healing and personal growth throughout this time in my life. I am grateful to have such wonderful peeps in my life.

CBD oils and products are being used for treatment of spinal cord injury/disease, arthritis, severe fibromyalgia, and anxiety secondary to post traumatic stress disorder, just to mention a few of the most common diagnoses/conditions that I have noticed respond well to CBD therapy. Also, I would like to mention the absolute miracles I have witnessed relating to cancer patients' success with CBD shrinking or correcting cellular balance of cancer tumors.

For example, a patient came into The CBD Store reporting she had seen the doctor here at the clinic and now she had been waiting more than 90 days to receive her Medical Cannabis Card from the State of Illinois to gain access and treat her stage III brain tumor which was not considered terminal according to the State of Illinois Medical Cannabis Pilot Program. She was asking what she could take along the lines of CBD that might assist with treating her brain tumor, or at least treating symptoms of pain and brain fog?

The store wellness specialist provided information about third party testing and I offered information about hemp healing properties, along with different routes and dosing suggestions obtained from reliable sources. Considering her other medications, and the fact that her food and fluid intake had decreased along with her appetite, the elderly lady/patient and I discussed several options on how much and how often to administer the CBD oil. (Note: throughout my hospice experience, I took notice that the size of the patient does not have anything to do with the dose size to meet pain control. e.g. some of my 100lb. female patients needed twice the amount of pain medication as the 200lb male patients to meet their reported pain control goals). Two weeks later, the same lady walked into The CBD Store reporting she had gone for her monthly checkup and had a scan that revealed the brain tumor was shrinking. The only change in her treatment plan was the administration of the miraculous CBD oil. We celebrated and shared happy tears and hugs -- one of my specialties. Final outcome success stories add to the reasons why we advocate, educate, and medicate with this amazing, safe, natural medicine.

Conversations with patients about their wellness journey and what has led them to seek CBD therapy often result in tears. 99 percent of the time, my experience has been listening to patients report they have exhausted traditional therapies and treatments. They are typically exhausted from trying everything known to man to treat their disease. They share openly that this is their last-ditch effort in treating their current symptoms and/or conditions. Patients report that their doctors have literally said there is nothing further to be done for them and have literally gone to the extent of giving a false prognosis, or even refusing to continue treating them at all.

After enduring months of expensive treatments and therapies with minimal relief from symptoms, coupled with opioid administration and, in some cases, addiction, these patients are facing exacerbated symptoms, resulting in more signs and symptoms of disease progression which also are not managed, so the cycle continues. Their stories are real and often heart-wrenching to listen to. These conversations would open a door of opportunity for me to provide education, validation of their chief complaints, and to listen to them talk about the inability to alleviate or reach symptom control goals and the range of emotions this brought on for them. Patients often report traditional treatment options have not served them well; this is when I often offer a hug, for I truly believe instilling hope, offering validation and support, and of course laughter can lead to a holistic approach in treating not only the body, but also the mind and spirit. Daily CBD oil, coupled with a little hope and love, go a long way.

For some, seeing is believing. Once they experience relief, coupled with a good understanding of the medication action and the science of the ECS, hemp as medicine is adding valuable quality to lives. I recall a male, middle-aged patient coming in to see Dr. C at our Pekin clinic. As he sat across from me, I pretty much had him assessed with my "nursing eyes" from across the room, as RNs' are trained to do. I noted he had facial grimacing and his mobility appeared very taxing. The patient reported he has had to ambulate with crutches for the past 3 years due to spinal issues. He had tried opioid treatment, trips to the pain clinic, and surgery; all failed to meet his pain management and symptom control goals. The patient also reported that he considers his stomach issues the result of long-term opioid use, which was encouraged by both his surgeon and primary-care physician, as well as the VA. After we discussed CBD education and I explained the stations-flow of the visit, I presented CBD med route deliveries, and with his permission, gave him a sample of the hemp topical butter/salve. After approximately 7 minutes, the patient smacked his hand on my desk and shouted, "I Do NOT Believe it -MY PAIN IS GONE!" We celebrated, and I counseled him about not over-doing it while feeling so great. He voiced his understanding, but he was so excited to express his idea that not needing his ambulation devices would add so much value to his quality of life. Shared moments like this with patients make my job so rewarding, words cannot express my gratitude for the peace the patients share. Patients will remember not only how they were treated, but the way we assisted them to feel and think about their approach to wellness and disease-process-treatment, and that there is hope.

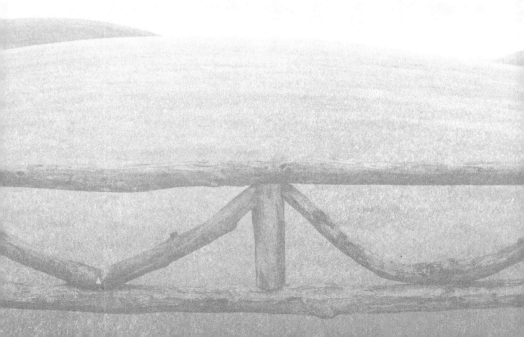

PART
Three

*"Science is a way of thinking much more
than it is a body of knowledge."*

—CARL SAGAN

Chapter

6

CANNABIS HAS BEEN USED MEDICINALLY for eons in numerous ancient cultures, including China, Egypt, Greece, and closer to home, many Native American tribes. Actually, at least one source we've read stated boldly that cannabis was used medicinally in ALL ancient cultures. The earliest documentation of cannabis being used for medicinal purposes comes from China, with the first record of its use as medicine in the *Pen-ts'ao ching*, the world's oldest book of medicinal drugs. The *Pen-ts'ao* is credited to Emperor Shen-Nung, who is recognized as the Father of Chinese Medicine. It lists more than 100 medical uses for cannabis.

Cannabis use naturally followed the trade routes, and by 1550 BCE an Egyptian papyrus of medical herbal knowledge, the *Ebers Papyrus*, noted cannabis was effective for treating inflammation. By 1200 BCE cannabis was being used medicinally in India, where it was revered as one of the five sacred plants in the Hindu sacred texts, the *Vedas*. In what is now the Middle East, records from Persian medicine traditions note the biphasic effects of cannabis, and Arabic medicine used cannabis to treat epilepsy. In the western hemisphere, many Native American tribes had practices that used cannabis for both rituals and medicine.

But the times have changed. Unfortunately, current cultures, including modern life in the US, have created obstacles for using this ancient remedy. Today we've all but forgotten how to use this hallowed botanical. Until very recently, cannabis plants, both hemp and marijuana, had been relegated to the status of vile, evil, illegal; and those who pursued cannabis as medicine despite its illegal status have been dubbed stoners and criminals. Luckily, the pendulum is swinging back, and at least since the passing of the 2018 Farm Bill, though truthfully a bit longer than that, people have been coming up with plentiful methods for using this ancient therapy. Some are better than others in terms of basing their products on supportive evidence their methodology is sound. Since the FDA hasn't yet issued guidelines as reference points, the market is unregulated, untamed, and full of loose information that may not be based on credible knowledge, experience, or insight; which is, at least potentially, a scary place. Unless or until the federal government creates standardized dosing guidelines for hemp-derived CBD, it is up to each person to develop a personal CBD protocol. Knowing how to get started and deciding how to proceed along the path are difficult and confusing for everyone.

WORK WITH YOUR DOCTOR!

The number of people using hemp-derived CBD products has grown exceptionally fast over the last few years, and this growth is expected to continue through the foreseeable future. Voters and politicians are both enthusiastically supporting legalization efforts as the market continues to expand. So far, though, doctors are not jumping on the bandwagon with the same fervor.

Very few doctors are prepared to make recommendations for hemp-derived CBD products to their patients. Most physicians don't have the same amount of knowledge and experience with Cannabis Medicine they have with traditional medicine because it is not included in medical school curricula. Plus, doctors cannot prescribe cannabis therapies; they are limited to simply making recommendations, which remains a pretty dark zone in the absence of federal guidelines. Despite this, we, and all credible resources for using CBD safely and appropriately, adamantly recommend working with your doctor to develop your personal CBD protocol.

As the CBD market and medical marijuana programs continue to grow, a few medical schools are beginning to offer some training in Cannabis Medicine. Additionally, training programs about Cannabis Medicine designed specifically for medical professionals, including doctors, are becoming available. In the meantime, many doctors remain not only hesitant, but truly opposed to recommending hemp-derived products for their patients. When asked about this reluctance, the answer is often something about inadequate supporting data based on clinical trials. We have been told that obtaining a blessing to proceed with research on Cannabis Medicine has not been easy because of its status as a Schedule 1 substance.

But in February of 2015, a doctor conducted a PubMed search for scientific journal articles published in the last 20 years containing the word "cannabis." The search revealed 8,637 results. When the word "cannabinoid" was added to the search, the results increased to 20,991 articles.[153] This hardly seems like a dearth of supporting data based on clinical trials. And that was 6 or 7 years ago, so it does not include any of the research conducted and reported since then.

So, doctors actually do have access to a large archive of supporting data based on clinical trials, and as more of them become interested in Cannabis Medicine and conduct their own searches, more doctors will be able to work with their patients who are interested in Cannabis Medicine. We envision a domino effect as physicians who are interested in learning as much as they can about Cannabis Medicine, and sharing this information with their colleagues, continue with their quest. As time goes on and research continues, presumably more and more doctors will become knowledgeable about Cannabis Medicine and therefore comfortable discussing it with their patients.

Another apparent obstacle for doctors with regard to supporting their patients' interest in using CBD is that, because of its lengthy incarceration as a Schedule 1 substance, many physicians are incorrectly under the impression they're not allowed to discuss CBD and other Cannabis Medicine options with their patients. They are mistakenly under the impression their license to prescribe pharmaceuticals could be jeopardized.

We find this fact particularly troublesome, considering hemp-derived CBD products, when produced in accordance with the law, became legal at the federal level in 2018. Many of the people we've spoken with have expressed how much they would appreciate being able to work with a doctor who could effectively blend traditional medicine with Cannabis Medicine. Considering the popularity of hemp-derived CBD products being used for health benefits, we believe it's imperative that physicians step up to the plate and honor the expanding expectation for medical professionals to stay well-informed and up-to-date on legal, effective options for their patients. There is no longer any valid reason for doctors to remain unprepared or unwilling to discuss and recommend CBD-based products for their patients.

But much earlier than 2018, the Ninth Circuit Court of Appeals ruled in the case *Conant v Walters (2002)* that physicians have a first amendment right to discuss Cannabis Medicine with their patients. The court ruled the federal government could not punish, nor threaten to punish, a doctor merely for discussing Cannabis Medicine with a patient.[154] Doctors can, and should be prepared to, discuss hemp-derived CBD products with their patients without worrying their license could be jeopardized. This case also highlights how the difference between hemp and marijuana has become critically important since hemp is now essentially legal at the federal level.

CYTOCHROME P450 ENZYMES

When developing a personal CBD protocol, inhibition of the Cytochrome P450 enzyme system (CYP450) is a critically important consideration for anyone who takes medication regularly, whether over-the-counter or prescription, or both. Just like grapefruit and grapefruit juice, CBD inhibits the function of the CYP450 enzymes, displacing chemical competitors and preventing these enzymes from metabolizing other compounds, like medications.

Metabolism is complicated; it relies on a huge number of biologic processes. Numerous molecular pathways and enzymes work together to break down compounds, which are then either used by the body or eliminated. CYP450 enzymes metabolize most medications by oxidizing them, or incorporating an oxygen atom into the medication's molecular structure, making it more water-soluble and easier for the kidneys to filter out. Certain levels of CBD will temporarily deactivate the CYP450 enzymes by occupying the site of enzymatic activity.

Some chemical compounds either induce or inhibit the CYP450 enzymes, creating interactions that could cause side effects. Inducers accelerate the rate of the other drugs' metabolism, reducing its effectiveness, which will likely prevent it from working as intended. Conversely, if a medication is taken with a substance that inhibits its metabolism, like CBD, the medication level can rise and possibly create harmful side effects. Knowing about the medications metabolized by CYP450 enzymes can help minimize the possibility of negative reactions and interactions. There is no minimum dose where CBD will not interact with other drugs.

Different methods of taking CBD have different effects; several variables affect the process, including how, and how much, CBD was taken. Other considerations include the individual characteristics of the person taking the CBD, and whether an isolate or a whole-plant product was taken. Inhaled CBD, whether smoked or vaped, enters the body through capillaries in the lungs, passes into general circulation through the pulmonary arteries, then quickly crosses the blood-brain barrier; the process is fast. However, when ingested orally, CBD is absorbed in the small intestine then delivered to the liver where it is metabolized by subclasses of CYP450 enzymes.

Some of the medications affected by CYP450 include:

- Antibiotics and antimicrobials,
- Anticancer medications,
- Antihistamines.
- Antiepileptic drugs (AEDs),
- Blood pressure medications,
- Blood thinners,
- Cholesterol medications,
- Corticosteroids,
- Erectile disfunction medications,
- GI medications, such as to treat GERD or nausea,
- Heart rhythm medications,
- Immunosuppressants,
- Mood medications, such as to treat anxiety, depression, or mood disorders,
- Pain medications,
- Prostate medications.[155]

Check the insert that comes with your medication for more information, or ask your doctor/pharmacist. Research to determine potential interactions between CBD and specific medications is ongoing, but in the meantime, there is a guiding principle to follow: *avoid CBD if your medication has a grapefruit warning.*

BIOAVAILABILITY

Another important issue to keep in mind when considering a personal CBD protocol is bioavailability, the amount or percentage of CBD actually absorbed into the bloodstream. The more that is actually absorbed, the stronger or more potent the effect will be. The main factors in determining CBD bioavailability are the type of CBD product consumed and the delivery method used.

Cannabinoids are lipophilic molecules, meaning they are oil-based compounds that are not soluble in water. This means that when extracted hemp oils are placed in water, they float. Cannabinoids, in their natural lipophilic state, do not mix with or dissolve in water, which is problematic because human bodies have difficulty absorbing these types of molecules. Taken orally, CBD has limited bioavailability, meaning only some of the CBD will make it all the way through the digestive system into the bloodstream. CBD bioavailability can be increased by taking it with a high-fat meal or snack, because CBD dissolves easily in fat and fatty oils that break down large CBD molecules into smaller ones, making them easier for the body to absorb.

POTENCY OR CONCENTRATION

CBD oil products are available in a variety of qualities and a range of strengths. There are seemingly endless different CBD manufacturers to choose from, and most offer products in at least two or three different potencies, or concentrations. By starting with the lowest potency, each person can effectively evaluate how much CBD they need to reach their goal. Many people, especially those who are new to cannabis, get a better result from a small amount of CBD than from a larger dose.

CBD is biphasic, meaning a little bit often delivers a bigger bang than a larger dose will; taking an excessive amount of CBD will probably be less effective than taking a moderate dose. So definitely start with the lowest potency and see if your goals are met. You can always bump it up if you're not accomplishing the results you were hoping for, but taking more than necessary to accomplish your goal will simply leave your body eliminating the excess. There is absolutely no benefit to taking more CBD than your body needs to accomplish your goals.

Always start with a small dose, especially if you have little or no experience with cannabis. The compounds in CBD oil often produce the opposite effects of what people expect; more is definitely not necessarily better. Although CBD is available in a wide range of concentrations, quality products provide between 250 mg and 5,000 mg per fluid ounce.

UNIVERSAL LAWS

There are a couple points that seem to be universal when it comes to figuring out the best ways to use CBD. One of the first "Universal Laws" is *Start Low and Go Slow*. We've heard this quote at least a million times, it seems, and read it almost as many. However, there is no standard for a starting point, or for how slowly to increase your dose, which is definitely confusing.

We have found that everybody in the industry, without exception, agrees with the mantra to start low and go slow, but there is a huge variation in what is considered starting low. The range of recommendations for starting a CBD protocol generally wavers between 15 mg and 50 mg per day. That's an incredibly huge variance, considering that, on the high end, the starting point is more than 3 times what the low one is, leaving consumers wondering why, and which is better? Another recommendation we've seen was to start at 6 mg per day for every 10 pounds of body weight, so a 200 lb. person would be starting at 120 mg, which is an incredibly high dose by all standards.

This is significant for several reasons, including the interesting fact that with CBD, more isn't necessarily better. Many people actually get a better result from CBD with a lower dose. And though people cannot "overdose" on CBD, negative side effects, while few and far between, are usually the result of over-consumption. Though it's generally well-tolerated, CBD has, on rare occasions, been known to cause mild side effects including dry mouth, diarrhea, reduced appetite, and drowsiness. Based on several of the recommendations we've seen, it seems like plenty of people should be in line for these negative side effects!

Regarding the second half of the mantra, to go slow, we've found similar results. Several sources recommend doubling your dosage daily until you feel better, others recommend doubling your dosage weekly. But none of them state an upper-end maximum. Apparently, they believe it is okay to simply continue doubling your dose until you feel better, regardless how long that takes or how high you end up going. If you're starting at 15 mg and double it daily, you'll be above 50 mg within just a few days, and if you start at 50, you'll be at a seriously high dose within a very short time. In our experience, 50 mg is a higher dose than most people can process or benefit from, and doses higher than 50 mg are rarely needed.

Furthermore, we did not find any credible sources offering guidance for addressing specific ailments, leaving consumers wondering why they would use the same protocol for their arthritis that their brother is using for his PTSD or a friend is using for her irritable bowel? Even well-informed people are left scratching their heads, feeling like they don't understand how to even get started on the journey to a personal CBD protocol.

There are a few web pages, generally for highly regarded and well-known medical establishments, that actually have charts with dosage recommendations for specific conditions. Although they each have a disclaimer saying something like, "The doctors at {such-and-such well-known clinic} have determined that the following doses are effective for the conditions listed," none of them provided any information explaining or supporting how the listed doses were determined. There was a fairly broad variation between them, leaving us, and all potential consumers, in the dark about why those particular doses made the chart, and most of them were extremely high. These recommendations definitely seemed contradictory to a conservative approach based on starting low and going slow.

Another "Universal Laws" is that the right dosage is highly personalized. Everyone is different, and each person responds to CBD in a unique, personalized way. There are countless variables, including each person's weight, diet, metabolism, genetics, environment, age, plus other variables like product consistency that all play a role in finding the dosage that works best for each individual.

A very important factor is whether or not the individual is taking medications, and if so, how many and how much, and for what condition(s). For example, if all other variables are the same, including body weight, someone who is taking a couple of medications to treat a couple of conditions will probably need a different dose of CBD than their identical twin who is lucky enough to not need any medications.

CBD AND METABOLISM

CBD has direct effects on human metabolism. By prompting the CB1 and CB2 receptors, it has the potential to help with metabolizing food during digestion. Homeostasis in the digestive process is critical for many reasons, including the fact that overstimulation of the ECS can lead to abdominal obesity, insulin resistance, and increased energy storage in fat cells.

Dictionary.com lists the definitions of Metabolism as:

1. *The sum of the physical and chemical processes in an organism by which its material substance is produced, maintained, and destroyed, and by which energy is made available,*

2. *Any basic process of organic functioning.*

Overstimulated CB1 receptors increase the chance of developing metabolic syndrome, a condition characterized by high blood sugar, high blood pressure, and excess body fat. According to researchers at the Endocannabinoid Research Group, since CBD is a CB1 antagonist, it could very likely have the ability to treat metabolic syndrome and other conditions like it.[156]

Medical researchers and doctors believe white fat increases the risk for several health conditions, including diabetes and heart disease, while brown fat potentially promotes weight loss by burning energy. In 2016, researchers published a study in the scientific journal *Molecular and Cellular Biochemistry* describing how they found CBD affects "fat browning" in three different ways:

1. CBD stimulates the proteins and genes involved with increasing the breakdown of fat.

2. CBD can boost the number and the activity of mitochondria, increasing the body's power to burn calories.

3. CBD reduces the expression of proteins involved in creating new fat cells.[157]

This research demonstrated CBD has the ability to induce "fat browning," or convert white fat into brown fat.

CLOSING THOUGHTS

Modern research is just beginning to catch up with much of the wisdom ancients learned with their own methods, however archaic their methods might seem compared to modern techniques. But modern researchers continue exploring how and why cannabinoid medicine works, and which conditions it manages well.

There are several things to consider once you're ready to begin a personal CBD protocol. One thing we definitely recommend is working with your doctor, though most doctors have limited knowledge and understanding about Cannabis Medicine. Remember, there is a pretty good chance you will be in a position to help your doctor learn about this growing field, but there are issues you should be prepared to discuss with your doctor, including how CBD might impact your prescribed medications. As time goes on, it is likely more and more doctors will be able to make informed recommendations for their patients who are interested in CBD therapy.

Determining the correct dose of CBD is an experiment for everyone. Because CBD is bi-phasic, most people actually get a better result from a small or moderate dose than a large one, including those who are bigger than average. The results of your CBD therapy will definitely be affected by your diet, your individual body weight and chemical makeup, and other factors, in addition to any medications you take. For this reason, always start with a low dose and increase it slowly in order to find your ideal dose without taking more than you need to reach your goals.

BOLD EXPLORERS
BLAZING THE TRAIL

"ON MY LAST CT SCAN, they found no evidence of cancer!"

These are the most amazing words a woman can say if that woman had been told her cancer was "incurable" and modern medicine might be able to help prolong her life, but could not offer her a cure.

Diagnosed with Metastatic Glioma Cell Carcinoma of the Vulva in November, 2017, Sheri has been undergoing regular chemo therapy treatments since then. Along with these treatments, she also takes an aggressive CBD therapy. Between the two, she has accomplished the miracle of "no evidence of cancer."

She credits this miraculous accomplishment to her amazing attitude. She believes every day is a good day to have a good day! She is quick to say that her mental and emotional strength are the combination that created the possibility of healing from her "incurable" cancer. Full of positivity and joy, even on the days when the side-effects from her chemo treatments leave her feeling pretty crummy, she says the CBD helps with the side-effects, and helps her maintain her positive attitude through it all.

Sometime about a year after she had started the chemo therapy, Sheri started on a CBD therapy to complement her chemo. Her CBD therapy includes using a tincture under the tongue, occasional edibles, and bath bombs. She explained that the bath bombs have been able to help ease the discomfort of her symptoms, the tincture is easy to use, and the edibles help with side-effects of the chemo like intestinal difficulties, plus the depression and anxiety that come with the cancer and cancer treatments.

She explains that her cancer doctors know she is taking CBD and have offered verbal support for her to continue with it, but they haven't expressed any real interest in her CBD therapy. They have not asked what she's taking, how she takes it, how she got started, how much she takes, or anything else. She is grateful her doctors haven't discouraged her from taking the CBD therapy, but thinks it would be amazing to have an oncologist who could effectively blend traditional chemo therapy treatments with CBD therapy.

Sheri – you are clearly a dreamer. Keep hoping for such an amazing advancement in medicine, and it just might happen! There are many people who share that hope and look forward to the day when Cannabis Medicine and traditional medicine are successfully blended to offer patients the best of both, including the synergy that can occur when they work together.

Until that time, keep up the good work! Not only are you a living, breathing miracle – you are an inspiration to others who have heard those devastating words from their own doctors. You've proven that "incurable" doesn't necessarily mean a death sentence. As more and more people are able to access Cannabis Medicine, the hope for cures to incurable diseases runs deep. You offer them a reason to continue down the path.

Thank you for blazing a trail in cancer care! And congratulations on your miraculous cure to an incurable disease!

Chapter

7

NO WONDER PEOPLE ARE CONFUSED about how to use CBD! Just getting started requires navigating something like a labyrinth of confusing information that, often enough, is as contradictory as the information about the health benefits of drinking coffee. Knowing who you can trust, and what information is valid is not easy. Figuring out how to take your CBD requires some trial and error for most people. But these things are important if you're going to get a positive result from a CBD regimen.

In this chapter you'll find information about how to get started on your own personal CBD protocol. Our recommendations are absolutely conservative with regard to starting low and going slow. Based on many years of helping many people who have been suffering from a vast spectrum of conditions, we have developed our recommendations to ease you into getting started without putting anyone at risk of developing negative consequences from over-consumption. Side effects from CBD are rare, but when they have happened, it has been in situations where people took more CBD than their body needed. Following the universal law of starting low and going slow is the best way to introduce your body to cannabinoids. Because CBD is biphasic, most people get a better result from a small or moderate dosage than they do from a larger one. Give yourself the best chance for the best outcome with this conservative strategy.

One important thing to keep in mind is that everyone's body is unique. Each person's ECS works according to their own metabolism and body chemistry, so a protocol that works really well for one person might not be a good match for someone else. Factors like your diet, relative health, and previous experience with cannabis all make a difference. The common idea that a big person will need a larger dose than a small person will to get a positive result just doesn't work with cannabinoids. We've seen some very large people get great results from surprisingly small dosages, and we've seen some tiny, wiry people with hardly any meat on their bones who needed a relatively large dose to accomplish their goals. With our recommendations, you can continue increasing your dosage incrementally as long as you need to, but you will give each incremental dosage a long enough try to know if you've actually reached the optimum level you need.

ESTABLISH YOUR CBD GOALS

The first step for anyone considering a CBD therapy regimen is to determine your personal goals for starting. What do you want to accomplish? What are you hoping the CBD will do for you? How will you know whether or not you've met your goal? How long are you willing to continue trying if you don't see the desired results quickly? What if you don't accomplish your desired goal, but feel like you are benefitting from the CBD therapy in other ways? What if you don't accomplish your desired goal and feel like you are not heading in the right direction – how long will you continue trying? You need to have some serious conversations with yourself about these kinds of questions, then discuss them with your doctors to determine when you're ready to get started.

START LOW AND GO SLOW

Once you've determined your baseline goals, be sure to start low and go slow! We recommend that everyone, regardless of other variables, starts with a very low dose of 5 mg daily for a period of at least one week. At the end of the first week, evaluate how you're feeling and how much closer you are to your goal. If you're not there yet, increase your daily dosage by the same amount, so you'll be taking 10 mg daily for another week. At the end of the second week, again evaluate how you're feeling. If you still haven't met your goal, continue increasing your dosage by the same amount for another week, and continue this pattern until you've reached your goal. Never increase your daily intake by more than this! Pay close attention to how you feel because some people get very dramatic results very quickly, but for others, the results are slower and more subtle.

There are a few people who do not even need 5 mg per day to reach and maintain their goals. If you start at the 5 mg dosage but feel a little groggy the next morning, try cutting back to just 2.5 mg for a week and see how you're feeling at this dosage. You can continue with the same strategy i.e. double your dose at the end of the first week, so that you're up to 5 mgs that following week. If you're still not meeting your goals, increase your intake by another 2.5 mgs. Most people who feel best starting at this lower dose do not end up needing very much, so again, pay very close attention to how you're feeling the first couple of weeks.

MICRO-DOSING

Another strategy we emphasize is micro-dosing, or spreading your daily intake out over small amounts taken several times each day. For example, if you are at the point of taking 25 mg of CBD per day, we suggest you take 5 mgs 5 times each day rather one full dose. If you're taking 50 mgs per day, try taking 10 mgs 5 times daily. This approach helps eliminate peaks and valleys in your systems.

A growing body of evidence indicates that spreading your dosage out over the course of the day by micro-dosing can increase the benefits from the CBD, regardless how much CBD you're taking. Cannabinoids are not like most treatments when it comes to finding the right dose. There is no such thing as a one-size-fits-all approach to CBD, but as the research with CBD continues to evolve, the evidence is pointing to factors that can affect the ways each individual's body responds to CBD. Different people benefit from different amounts of CBD than others, even if their health status and concerns are similar. Ultimately, though, the goal of micro-dosing is to supply the body with a steady stream of plant cannabinoids, helping you maintain balance.

OPTIONS FOR TAKING CBD

People are definitely coming up with plentiful methods for using this ancient therapy. Deciding which method(s) you'd like to get started with is one of the first questions you'll need to answer once you decide you're ready to give CBD a try. You will definitely need to explore which delivery method best suits you personally; there is no method of taking CBD that suits all users. CBD is available in a variety of forms with numerous different concentrations.

The method you choose for taking CBD will depend on your personal goals and lifestyle. For example, if you're looking for the best option to help manage anxiety, you will probably want to try a fast-acting method. If one of your goals is to manage chronic inflammation, you're likely to want a method that stays in your system for a while. Other considerations include whether you need to be discrete about taking the product, and how picky you are about taste and texture.

Depending on your personal goals and preferences, there are numerous delivery methods to choose from. For each person, finding the right product can take some patience and curiosity, as the one you try first might not seem to work for you. But don't despair; there is sure to be at least one delivery method that will work for you. Once you've decided on the delivery method you're interested to try, you will need to assess the concentration of CBD in the actual product before knowing how much to use.

Plan to take your first dose in the evening, an hour or two before you go to bed. Take your CBD, then take a shower or bath, so you are relaxed, and then put on your favorite Netflix or read a good book. Don't drink alcohol. The point is to pay close attention to how the CBD makes you feel, so you don't want to complicate it with other substances. Also, don't take sleeping pills. CBD works well for easing insomnia, and you don't want your CBD experience to be clouded by the effects of a sleep enhancement therapy.

Always take your first dose on the weekend, or on an evening that it won't complicate your life if you're not feeling 100% the next morning. Most people feel just fine in the morning, but a few people feel a bit groggy. If you're one of the few who feels a little groggy in the morning, take a smaller dose the next night and then re-evaluate how you feel the next morning.

Oral Delivery

Capsules are one of the most popular CBD delivery options. If you're new to CBD, ingesting capsules is an easy way to get started. Monitoring your dosage is easy with capsules since they come in pre-measured sizes. Having a consistent concentration makes it easier to find out what actually works well for you. CBD soft gels are infused with the same CBD oil available in tinctures, and they have several advantages, including how easy they are to take and the fact you get an accurate and consistent amount with each capsule.

Edibles are another popular option. A CBD gummy is simply a gummy candy infused with CBD. Options for edibles usually include candy like gummies, chocolate bars, and hard candies, plus pastry items like cookies and brownies, and a variety of other treats, depending on where you purchase your CBD. They're easy to take because the dose is pre-measured, and they can be taken anywhere. You can make your own edibles at home if you are inclined; there are plenty of recipes online.

Chewing Gum is one of the easiest, most efficient, and tasty ways to add CBD to a wellness routine. Gum releases the CBD directly into the blood-stream through the membranes of the mouth and throat, so delivery is fast, and the bioavailability is better than with most other oral delivery methods. People in recovery from substance abuse often find chewing gum provides a rhythmic distraction to focus on instead of cravings.

Tinctures in dropper-bottles are one of the most popular delivery methods for CBD oil. They are easy for beginners to use and also a favorite with people who've been using CBD for some time. Tinctures are available in a variety of strengths and flavors. The droppers are marked with measurements, so it's easy to get a fairly precise dose, making tinctures one of the easiest methods for experimenting with different strengths. Once you've got your dose in the dropper, simply squirt it under your tongue and hold it for 30 – 60 seconds. This method is fast-acting and effective.

Everybody knows oil and water don't mix very well, so beverage makers are faced with a fundamental challenge when trying to mix CBD with beverages: it is insoluble. However, there are now water-soluble products on the market, and one of those will be best if you want to add CBD to your coffee or tea, lemonade, juice, smoothies, or even in a glass of water. The oil is converted into a water-soluble powder, then broken down into micro-sized droplets of oil that are encapsulated within other non-toxic materials so that they remain stable. The end result of this process is an off-white, water-soluble, micro-encapsulated, hemp CBD extract. The conversion process allows CBD oil to be consumed orally without sacrificing bioavailability.

Inhaled Delivery

Vapes are a popular method for taking CBD. Vaping is simple, so it's easy to use, but it is definitely not a good fit for everyone. CBD made for vaping is sometimes called "CBD vape oil," but it doesn't contain any actual oil; a more appropriate name would be "CBD vape juice." Vape cartridges are available in a range of flavors and strengths, and they're generally made with food grade ingredients, but don't be fooled – they are very different from oil-based tinctures.

Look carefully at the ingredients. If you see anything listed other than PG, VG, CBD extract, terpenes, and cannabinoids, then it's probably not suitable for inhalation. Don't take the risk. The label should indicate, in some way, something about vaping, vape juice, e-liquid, or e-juice, and should not list any actual oil among the contents. CBD cartridges are slim, disposable e-cig tanks filled with CBD e-juice that connect to a standard 510 thread battery. There are also cartridges, known as pods, compatible with popular vape equipment. Vaping is one of the fastest-acting delivery methods, so it is really useful for issues like anxiety when a quick result is important.

Smoking hemp buds is another way for people to inhale CBD. Hemp buds can be smoked exactly the way marijuana buds are smoked. The difference is that smoking hemp buds will not produce the "high" that smoking marijuana is known for. Smoking hemp flower is one of the most effective ways to experience the benefits of CBD. The primary concern for people who prefer smoking is the potential long-term effects on the lungs.

Inhalation is an effective delivery method for CBD because of how quickly it absorbs into the body. When CBD is smoked or vaped, cannabinoids are introduced directly to the lungs and then rapidly absorbed into the bloodstream and begin circulating throughout the body, reaching peak concentration within minutes. Inhaling is a very efficient way to maximize bioavailability.

Topical Delivery

CBD-infused topicals include lotions, salves, and creams. In order for these products to penetrate lower layers of the skin, they must be transdermal so that active ingredients are absorbed into the circulatory system. The key benefits of CBD topicals include reducing pain and inflammation, soothing skin problems, and helping wounds heal. Topical CBD is also being used to successfully ease a variety of skin diseases, including some skin cancers. Topicals are available in a variety of strengths. Getting the proper dose of CBD through the skin may not be as straightforward as simply applying a moisturizer; it's important to find out how many milligrams of CBD are in the product in order to know if there is enough CBD to provide therapeutic relief.

In addition to massaging CBD topicals into the area of the body experiencing pain and/or inflammation, there is an ancient Indian tradition, Ayurveda, which focuses on connections between physical and spiritual health. An ancient Ayurvedic philosophy emphasizes the navel as a powerhouse of the human body. According to this tradition, oiling the belly-button with different types of oil, including CBD, has a variety of health benefits. In Ayurvedic medicine, a gland called the Pechoti sits behind the navel and allows humans to absorb substances like CBD oil into the body. This belief is based on the idea that humans absorb nutrients through the navel tissues and the umbilical cord when in the womb, so these same tissues will transport oils and other nutrients after birth.

Another, more traditional idea related to the Pechoti method appears to have Western research behind it, stating that nerves in the gut contain CB2 receptors allowing CBD oils to help with digestion.

CBD patches represent another method of topical delivery. Currently, there are two types of CBD patches on the market: matrix patches and reservoir patches. Matrix patches usually contain five layers: a peel-off layer that protects the CBD, a "matrix" layer infused with CBD, a separating layer, an adhesive layer that holds the matrix layer in place on the skin, and a protective backing layer. The CBD molecules move from the patch directly into the bloodstream. Transdermal patches are very similar to nicotine or birth control patches, with a few innovative twists to ensure the patch effectively delivers CBD to the bloodstream. They contain a measured dose of CBD, typically infused in an isolated solution, gel, or oil. Combined with carriers and permeation enhancers, the patch's high concentration of CBD coupled with skin's low concentration of CB1 receptors helps move the cannabinoids out of the patch and into the body.

Reservoir patches are different in important ways. They still have a peel-off layer, an adhesive, and a protective backing, but the key element is a permeable release membrane. Manufacturers can fine-tune the membrane to control the pace and rate of CBD delivery, so the patch releases CBD at a steadier, more controlled pace, rather than the tapered release of a matrix patch.

CBD patches deliver cannabinoids directly into the bloodstream and the ECS with minimal loss along the way. As a bonus, CBD also activates the skin cells directly, which can be beneficial for people with skin disorders. CBD patches are one of the most discreet delivery options that steadily release cannabinoids into the body over time.

Another method offering effective CBD delivery are suppositories. They provide a safe alternative for people who struggle with capsules or have a heightened gag reflex, or who are experiencing restricted oral intake before and after surgery. Suppositories offer an alternative delivery method when people are sick and vomiting, or have suffered an injury to the jaw or throat, or are dealing with various gastrointestinal challenges. Because suppositories bypass both the digestive and respiratory systems, CBD reaches the bloodstream in much higher concentrations. CBD suppositories are formulated for many uses, including relief during menstruation, or for targeted muscular relaxation and inflammation relief. These products can be used vaginally or rectally.

Additionally, CBD products have made their way into the bedroom. Found in a variety of products aimed at helping improve users' sex lives, these CBD products include personal lubricants, massage lotions, oral sprays, and edibles, as well as suppositories. Early research has CBD enthusiasts excited about the potential these products bring for both health and sexuality, though so far, most experts agree more studies are needed before any firm conclusions can be drawn. However, healthcare professionals say they've seen improvements in patients' sex lives, and anecdotal evidence has them convinced these CBD products are effective.

Another option for taking CBD are bath bombs and bath salts. These products typically contain CBD oil combined with essential oils and fragrances. There is minimal scientific research exploring the specific benefits of CBD bath bombs and bath salts, but a closer look at the research exploring the benefits of CBD on the skin can explain the potential benefits of bath bombs and salts. Manufacturers of these products tend to state they provide psychological and skin benefits.

These are some of the most popular ways of taking CBD, but new delivery methods are being tested and introduced regularly. Keep your eyes and ears open to stay apprised as new products and product-categories become available.

GETTING OFF TRADITIONAL/ PHARMACEUTICAL MEDICATION(S)

One of the main goals many clients come to us with is getting off their pharmaceutical medications. If this is one of your goals, or your main goal, try our protocol of starting with a very small amount of CBD, increasing slowly in incremental amounts for a few weeks to see how you respond to it, then consider cutting your dosage of pharmaceuticals back in incremental steps while simultaneously increasing your CBD by small, incremental doses. Using this strategy, we have been able to help at least 75% of our clients accomplish their goal of either cutting back on their medications or eliminating them completely. But it takes time and patience.

At one point, we were working with 8 individuals who had been diagnosed with Stage IV cancer (terminal), but wanted to get off of their medications. Following our protocol, 6 of the 8 were successful at both getting off of their harmful cancer medications and surviving! The daughter of one of the others contacted us after her mother had passed and shared that, though she had not survived, her mother had been able to enjoy her last days. With the CBD therapy, she had been able to eat, sleep, and laugh; all things she had not been able to do when taking only her traditional treatments. The daughter felt the CBD therapy greatly improved her mother's final days.

CLOSING THOUGHTS

Getting started with a personal CBD protocol is an experiment for everyone, but the results can be tremendous! Cannabis Medicine has been practiced for centuries, and now, after a lengthy hiatus of being criminalized, it is currently experiencing a renaissance that allows people to partake of the benefits this natural plant remedy offers.

There are now several varieties of CBD oil products available, and variations on how much and how many of the cannabinoids people take, as well. CBD has direct effects on human metabolism by prompting the CB1 and CB2 receptors, and though there are some potential challenges to using it safely with certain pharmaceuticals, it has proven to be a very effective preventive therapy for numerous health conditions. Though most doctors don't yet feel prepared or comfortable to make recommendations to their patients who are interested in Cannabis Medicine, the tides are beginning to turn.

The extensive variety of delivery options can seem overwhelming, but with a little patience and persistence, each person can find at least one delivery method that works for them. Implementing our methodology of starting low, increasing slowly, and micro-dosing is a sure thing for almost everyone, regardless of other variables in personal circumstances, allowing each person to feel confident about defining their personal CBD protocol.

BOLD EXPLORERS
BLAZING THE TRAIL

EILEEN STARTED HAVING SEIZURES in her late 50s. She hadn't been feeling well for several months. She described being tired all the time. It didn't matter how much sleep she had gotten, she never felt rested. But getting a good night's sleep was nothing more than a dream, because insomnia was haunting her. Then the headaches started, and they quickly became migraines. And the migraines continually got worse, each one more intense than the one before it, lasting longer, coming faster and faster. Then she had her first seizure, a grand mal seizure that lasted several minutes.

Turns out she had a benign brain tumor that was growing quickly. She underwent surgery to remove the tumor and the migraines stopped, but she continued having seizures. She began having panic attacks because of her fear and anxiety about the seizure activity escalating. Her panic attacks got to the point they were as much of a problem for her as the seizures.

She then experienced something like a downward spiral as she became intertwined in the series of seizures and panic attacks. Her doctors had her taking quite a few medications to control her seizure activity, her migraines, her anxiety, and to (hopefully!) prevent the tumor from coming back. Each of these medications had side effects, and she felt like a zombie all the time. Her fatigue never ended. Needless to say, she sank deeper and deeper into a dark hole of depression.

Eileen was at a loss. Her condition was having negative effects in every aspect of her life. Her adult children wanted her to quit her job, though she felt like the job was the only thing offering her a light on the horizon. She felt like the question of quitting her job was not even a consideration because now, more than ever, she needed her health insurance. Her husband worried about her to the extent it was having negative effects on his performance at work.

Her husband had heard enough about CBD that he was interested to learn more about it, hoping it might be a miracle solution for Eileen. Like so many people, neither of them had any idea how to get started, or who could give them trustworthy information. When he came to us seeking some advice, he was at his wits end, having been told a variety of conflicting things from a few different CBD shops. Rather than feeling like they helped him understand how to get started, he was completely confused and overwhelmed.

We helped Eileen get started on a very low-dose broad spectrum tincture, as she felt strongly about staying away from THC because of her job, and a fast-acting vape to use when she felt her anxiety kicking in.

She was thrilled that her seizures diminished immediately, but they didn't completely stop. She was excited to try a larger dose, and was disappointed when we discouraged her from doing that. Rather, we encouraged her to go slow and only increase her dosage by small increments week after week. To her credit, she listened, and after just a couple weeks following our protocol, her seizure activity had cut back to the point they were almost gone.

Following our protocol, Eileen has successfully gotten off most of her medications, and has been able to cut back on the two she continues taking. She has had no more tumors, and has been able to keep her job. Her migraines have subsided, she continues having only a few very minor seizures, and she is steadily regaining her strength. She says the CBD helps with her insomnia, and getting some sleep helps with her depression. Her anxiety and depression are both better, and she is able to enjoy most of the activities she enjoyed before the tumor, the headaches, the migraines, and the seizures. She states boldly the CBD helps with all of these issues. Eileen tells us the CBD gave her life back!

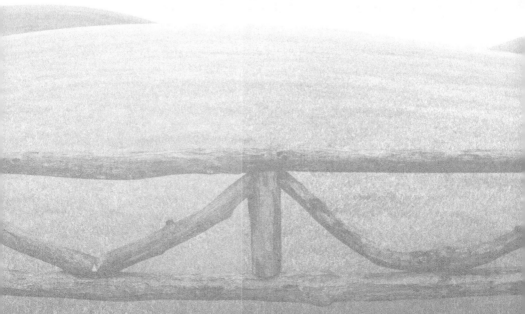

PART
Four

"It's amazing how a little tomorrow can make up for a whole lot of yesterday."

—JOHN GUARE

Chapter

8

IN THE FEW SHORT YEARS since the 2018 Farm Bill was passed, the hemp/CBD industry has changed dramatically. Despite what seem like enormous odds, including an ongoing effort to legalize marijuana at the federal level, the global pandemic and its accompanying economic disruptions, severely compromised supply chains, and inflation skyrocketing out-of-control, the hemp/CBD market is expected to continue growing at an astounding rate over the next several years. CBD sales in the US hit $4.6 billion in 2020, a colossal number just two years after federal legalization, and this breakneck growth is expected to continue. Forecasts are projecting a US market of $20 billion by 2025. As demand for CBD continues to grow, the industry is also creating jobs. There were an estimated 321,000 full-time jobs in the cannabis industry in 2020, up from 234,700 in 2019.[158] As the hemp/CBD job market continues to mature, the industry is creating its own definitions of what it takes to be successful in the market place. Labor economists say the industry is being defined by a priority to create favorable working conditions, both to attract employees and to gain broader legitimacy. Some employers feel compelled to treat their staff particularly well, given the uncertainty of working in an industry that remains dubious at the federal level. Working in the cannabis industry is not without risks.

WHO IS CAUSING ALL THE COMMOTION?

Who are the customers driving this phenomenal growth? Many analysts automatically expect the Millennial generation to be the market leader, but Baby Boomers are using CBD in surprisingly large numbers. In 2018, a little over 8% of Baby Boomers said they used CBD, more than any other age group at that time.[159] A 2019 Gallup poll showed women were more likely to use CBD products than men, making female Baby Boomers the most common CBD users in America.[160] But the CBD market continues evolving in response to changing demand, and in the current market (December, 2021), Millennials and Gen Xers make up a significant portion of CBD users (71%).[161] A large percentage of both generations said they use CBD daily. Millennials claim to take more doses per day, and people in both of these generations are more knowledgeable about CBD dosing than Baby Boomers. And though most of the members of Generation Z aren't old enough to buy cannabis products, those who are already make up a strong consumer group. In the first half of 2021, Gen Z overtook Baby Boomers with more cannabis sales for the first time ever, and this trend is likely to continue.

Despite its phenomenal growth, the CBD market has definitely not been immune to the economic impacts of COVID-19. As the world continues grappling with the pandemic, members of the hemp/CBD industry have had to scramble in a business environment that was already changing quickly. Entire marketing and sales strategies toppled because of conditions like stores closing and consumer purchasing patterns changing. E-commerce has become the dominant sales channel, with online CBD sales accounting for at least 60% of sales.[162] As the pandemic and its effects on the hemp/CBD market continue, changes will continue to unfold. Some trends the hemp/ CBD market is expected to experience over the next few years include:

- Higher potency products,
- Expanded online access,
- Increased pharmaceutical CBD products.

This last point, that more pharmaceutical CBD products are expected in the coming years, is likely to drive the most significant changes in the market.

BIG PHARMA ENTERS THE PICTURE

At the beginning of Chapter 1, we mentioned a 2019 study published in *the Hemp Business Journal* predicting sales of CBD products would continue to grow at an unprecedented rate, and the pharmaceutical industry would become the leader. This is unfolding exactly as predicted. For example, in spite of patent #6630507 having only one license associated with it, issued to Kannalife Sciences, another company, GW Pharmaceuticals (known in the US as Greenwich Biosciences), completed a new drug application for Epidiolex in 2017 and received FDA approval to treat pediatric epilepsy in June 2018. Analysts at Goldman Sachs predicted that Epidiolex will earn more than $2.2 billion a year by 2025, and that's just one CBD-based medication. Imagine how much money is likely to be earned with the contract Kannalife secured through patent #6630507. It's a lot!

In an effort to garner as much of the colossal amounts of money to be earned in the hemp/CBD market as possible, Big Pharma has been working to prevent the legal cannabis market from expanding. For example, in 2016 the drug manufacturer Insys Therapeutics made the largest campaign donation against Arizona's recreational marijuana initiative, with the result that Arizona was the only state where the initiative didn't pass. Insys Therapeutics opposed legalization because, at the time, they were getting ready to launch their new drug, Syndros, a synthetic version of THC. By donating a huge amount of money -- substantial enough to effectively alter the outcome of the election -- Big Pharma was able to quash the initiative that would have created competition for their synthetic version of the exact product they were actively opposing. Ironies abound in the CBD market! It's no surprise that Insys's latest drug is a synthetic version of CBD.

However, synthetic cannabinoid products are more potent and dangerous than natural, full spectrum cannabis products. They are known to induce severe adverse side effects, including respiratory difficulties, hypertension, chest pain, muscle twitches, renal failure, anxiety, agitation, psychosis, suicidal ideation, and cognitive impairment. Chronic use of synthetic cannabinoids has been associated with serious psychiatric and medical conditions, and even death.[163]

But synthetic cannabinoid products aren't the only pharmaceutical drugs facing financial issues with the possible legalization of cannabis. A study by *Bradford and Bradford* found in states where medical marijuana has been legalized, prescriptions for drugs effectively replaced with cannabis-based products decreased substantially. Big Pharma is moving into the cannabis market in other ways, as well. Early in 2021 a global biopharma company, Jazz Pharmaceuticals, bought GW Pharmaceuticals, the maker of Epidiolex, for $7.2 billion. Announced on February 3, 2021, the acquisition of GW by Jazz was characterized as the most significant foray by a drug company into the cannabis arena to date. Then in December 2021, pharmaceutical giant Pfizer Inc. entered the cannabis market with a $6.7 billion acquisition of Arena Pharmaceuticals, Inc., a biotech company with a segment dedicated to cannabinoid therapies. The core of Arena's cannabinoid program is research and development of an investigational drug, Olorinab, an oral full agonist of CB2 receptors being developed to treat pain associated with gastrointestinal disease. More than 100 drug companies are testing numerous new products based on synthetic versions of CBD and other cannabinoids, indicating cannabis-based drugs are quickly becoming legitimate within the pharmaceutical industry.

Big Pharma has begun lobbying the FDA to reschedule cannabis off of Schedule 1, much like cannabis advocates have been doing for decades. In this case, though, the reason is that rescheduling would allow the combination of the FDA, doctors, and pharmaceutical companies to control the production, prescription, and distribution of these products, paving the way for complete pharmaceutical regulation. Many people in the hemp/CBD industry believe Big Pharma will continue seeping into the market and that they will ultimately dominate it. As time goes on, when you hear about increasing restrictions on medical cannabis, pay attention to who is funding it, and don't be surprised when it is Big Pharma.

WHAT ABOUT LEGALIZATION?

Attitudes surrounding Cannabis Medicine are changing quickly in other arenas, as well. A debate about whether cannabis should be legalized has been lively for decades, and it is currently receiving a tremendous amount of attention in Congress. Federal legalization would disrupt the current patchwork of state-legal marijuana markets, creating the opportunity for interstate trade and the formation of regional (and national?) cannabis markets.

During the months leading up to the 2020 election, members of Congress had introduced several bills aimed at decriminalizing or otherwise loosening federal restrictions on cannabis. These included the STATES Act, a bill introduced in June 2018 to ensure every state can independently decide the best legal policies toward cannabis within its borders. Because cannabis remains an illegal substance at the federal level, it is still considered a felony to produce, distribute, or use marijuana, even though many states allow its use for medical purposes, and several states have legal recreational programs. The STATES Act does not propose legalizing cannabis at the federal level, but instead proposes to protect individuals and companies working in compliance with state laws where they differ from federal laws. If passed, the STATES Act will amend the Controlled Substances Act so state-compliant cannabis businesses will not be in violation of federal law. Rather than forcing states to legalize cannabis, the STATES Act would have cannabis remain illegal in states where it is currently illegal unless that situation changes through each individual state's legislative process.

Another bill before Congress is the MORE Act, which would decriminalize cannabis and expunge criminal records for nonviolent cannabis-related crimes. This act passed with a 24–10 majority by the House Judiciary Committee following markup on November 20, 2019. Two Republicans voted in favor of it, making this the first time in history a congressional committee approved a bill to end federal marijuana prohibition. The MORE Act would create a federal tax on marijuana with the revenue allocated to community reinvestment programs.

In July of 2021, Senate Majority Leader, Chuck Schumer, and two of his colleagues introduced a bill to legalize and regulate cannabis at the federal level, titled "The Cannabis Administration and Opportunity Act." This bill would:

- Remove marijuana and THC from the Controlled Substances Act.
- Transfer agency jurisdiction over cannabis from the DEA to a coalition made up of the FDA, the Alcohol and Tobacco Tax and Trade Bureau, and the Bureau of Alcohol, Tobacco, Firearms, and Explosives.
- Allow cannabis products to be transported across state lines, including through states where cannabis is illegal.
- Impose a federal excise tax on the sale of cultivated marijuana – 10% of the removal price for the first year, followed by annual increases up to 25% over the next three years. (Removal price is the price of the sale from cultivator to any third party.)
- Establish a trust fund and transfer the greater of either $10 million or 10% of the annual excise tax collected on cannabis. The fund would be managed by the Small Business Administration and be used for loans to women and historically socially and economically

disadvantaged individuals to be used in connection with the recipient's cannabis business.

- Establish and conduct a study into the impacts of driving under the influence of marijuana.
- Establish and conduct a study into the impacts of cannabis use on the human brain and the efficacy of cannabis use for medical purposes.
- Develop federal advertising regulations to prevent marketing to children and young adults.
- Provide funding to states to be used for expunging convictions of state level marijuana crimes.

As another reminder of how strong the push for legalization really is, in November of 2021, a freshman Republican from South Carolina introduced a bill to federally legalize and tax marijuana as an alternative to the pending Democratic-led reform proposals. This bill would take specific steps to ensure businesses in existing state markets are able to continue operating, regardless of changing federal rules. This legislation represents an attempt to bridge the partisan divide by incorporating certain equity provisions like expungements for people with non-violent cannabis convictions, and imposing an excise tax that would support community reinvestment, law enforcement, and Small Business Administration activities. This new enthusiasm from a Republican lawmaker representing a red state just might be the jump-start needed to move the bill forward.

At any other time in history, these bills would probably not receive legitimate consideration, but at this time, federal legalization has been introduced by members of both parties, including the Senate Majority Leader who has support from dozens of law makers. Regardless whether any of these bills passes or not, the idea of legalizing cannabis at the federal level is no longer the crazy notion it has been in the past. Most people believe it is no longer a question of "If" legalization will happen, but "When?"

GUIDELINES, ANYONE?

Although hemp and hemp-derived products like CBD were basically legalized by the 2018 Farm Bill, the FDA has yet to develop a process allowing derivatives like CBD to be used in products like foods, drinks, and dietary supplements. As a department of the US federal government, the role the FDA plays is to ensure the things we eat and drink, and the medications we take, are safe and effective. But where Cannabis Medicine is concerned, there seems to be a distorted vision of what this responsibility actually means and to whom they are responsible. According to the FDA, because CBD has been studied and approved as a drug, it cannot be considered a dietary supplement, and this has become a problematic issue.

At the time of this writing (December, 2021), three years have come and gone since the 2018 Farm Bill was signed into law, yet the FDA hasn't yet developed guidelines to regulate hemp-derived extracts. Rather, the FDA maintains the position that it is illegal:

> "... to introduce or deliver for introduction into interstate commerce any food (including any animal food or feed) to which has been added a substance which is an active ingredient in a drug product that has been approved under section 505 of the FD&C Act [21 USC § 355], or a drug for which substantial clinical investigations have been instituted and for which the existence of such investigations has been made public."[164]

This prohibition applies to CBD, they say, because it is an active ingredient in at least one known drug product, Epidiolex, that has been approved under section 505 of the FD&C Act.

The FDA had been promising to explore a regulatory pathway for the retail sale of hemp-derived CBD when they announced in October of 2021 that they don't plan to create such regulations any time soon. Acting Commissioner, Janet Woodcock, argued that current law is fairly clear in barring the agency from action on CBD, placing the FDA in a stalemate position. She went on to say she doesn't believe the question of the FDA developing guidelines for CBD is a matter of FDA policy, but a matter of law.

While plenty of people disagree with her interpretation, this stance has left many people feeling like congressional action is the only way to "stop the stalemate and regulate CBD now," a phrase that became the theme of a campaign launched by a coalition of hemp companies, organizations, and consumer groups advocating for federal legislation to establish a regulatory framework for retail sales of CBD products.

There are currently (December, 2021) three bills before Congress that would establish federal regulations for the sale of CBD products:

- H.R. 841 would regulate CBD as a dietary supplement.
- The CBD Product Safety and Standardization Act would establish federal standards and require the FDA to regulate CBD in foods and beverages.
- S 1698 would explicitly legalize CBD products in dietary supplements plus food and beverages.

Uncertainty surrounding the question of regulating CBD products has driven a sharp decline in hemp prices, resulting in economic hardship for hemp farmers. In the meantime, scores of CBD products are being sold with some of them continuing to raise serious concerns about potency, quality, safety, and other consumer protection issues. This obviously tarnishes the industry for all of the legitimate businesses operating within the law. Many people believe having some form of government oversight regulating CBD-based products as dietary supplements and food additives would provide guidance for the industry, protect consumers, and further legitimize the industry. Since the FDA continues declining to offer guidance, it's beginning to look like Congress is next in line to step up to the plate.

WHAT DOES THE RESEARCH SAY?

While the questions of if and when cannabis will become legalized at the federal level remain to be answered, and the question of who will bite the bullet and actually define guidelines for hemp/CBD products awaits an answer, other legislative changes have opened the doors for more human clinical trials. Researchers are investigating the effects CBD could have with a whole spectrum of conditions including autism, chronic pain, mood disorders, alcohol and other addictions, Crohn's disease, arthritis, cancer, and many others. The range of conditions CBD is being researched for seems awfully wide, but we already know CBD has far-reaching physiological effects, and increasing our understanding of how they can best be used remains a puzzle in many circumstances.

More than 20 mechanisms of action for CBD have already been identified. The effects resulting from such a broad range of actions are clearly exciting, and they absolutely justify consideration of a wide range of possible therapeutic uses. For example, CBD seems to effectively prevent seizure activity by binding to a protein that can trigger seizures by promoting hyperactivation of neurons. Additionally, CBD is known to act on receptors that mediate pain signaling and inflammation, and it acts on at least one receptor for the neurotransmitter serotonin. Exciting progress is being made toward easing many conditions that tend to be very difficult to treat effectively, yet they affect huge numbers of people. Scores of people are in line to benefit from ongoing research about the medical potential for CBD.

Mental Health represents one of the most promising areas for CBD research. In 1995, researchers reported the case of a person living with schizophrenia who experienced meaningful relief from their symptoms when treated with CBD. Several subsequent small-scale clinical studies have demonstrated similar results. In one study, treatment with CBD was associated with elevated levels of the endocannabinoid anandamide, which appears to help prevent psychosis.[165] In other research, scientists conducted a randomized controlled trial that showed CBD can help people who are using traditional anti-psychotic medications. When CBD was used hand-in-hand with conventional anti-psychotic treatments, patients experienced better symptom control of issues like hallucinations and delusions than with conventional treatments alone.[166]

Anxiety disorders are another mental-health condition CBD has been shown to help manage. Researchers used a test that simulated speaking in public to demonstrate how using a single dose of CBD before beginning to speak successfully reduced nervousness and discomfort in people with social anxiety disorder.[167] A similar effect has been observed with healthy people in anxiety-inducing situations, and several researchers are exploring CBD as a means of soothing social stress for people living with autism spectrum disorder (ASD). Many patients living with ASD are also diagnosed with epilepsy, and clinical trials are exploring how CBD can offer meaningful therapy for these patients.

And though cannabis has been demonized as a gateway drug leading users to experiment with more dangerous substances, research has actually demonstrated it contains an effective antidote for potentially deadly addictions. After observing rats with heroin addictions becoming less likely to seek out the opioid when treated with CBD, researchers started investigating whether CBD might have the same effects on people living with opioid dependency. Study participants who were given CBD reported lower levels of drug cravings and anxiety, and they reported the beneficial effects lasted for at least a week after taking the final dose of CBD.[168] These results are promising and offer at least a glimmer of hope for people battling addictions.

The amount of research being conducted around CBD and its potential therapeutic uses is huge – much too large to give any real credit and attention here. We chose to highlight the significant potential CBD is demonstrating with mental health conditions because CBD works differently than traditional treatments. With a different mechanism of action to dopamine receptor antagonists than standard medications, which have been the mainstay treatment of mental health disorders since the 1950s, CBD represent a completely different class of anti-psychotic treatment. As we discussed in the introduction, we are all living through a period of time that is really challenging, and plenty of people are trying to navigate these difficult times while managing anxiety and depression. CBD has helped a lot of people who live with these issues.

And if living through the pandemic somehow isn't enough of a challenge, the opioid crisis rages on, as well as alcoholism and plenty of other addictions. Knowing that CBD helps with cravings and anxiety will absolutely prove to be a strong weapon in the arsenal of tools for helping people live through the challenges of addiction. And finally, to imagine people who are living with debilitating psychoses being able to better manage their diseases is truly amazing, and being able to do so without side-effects is even better. CBD has the potential to make living with mental illness different, and seemingly better.

HEADLINE NEWS!

Research related to cannabis is continuing and expanding at unprecedented rates. During the past week while we've been preparing this chapter, a number and variety of research-related headlines have crossed our desks, and we've listed several of them here just to prove the point:

- Cannabis And Covid: Cannabinoid Acids Found In Hemp Can Prevent And Treat Coronavirus Infection, New Research Suggests,
- THIS TERPENE MAKES PAIN RELIEF BETTER AND WORSE, VIA THE CB1 RECEPTOR,
- Israeli cannabis start-up leads the way in killing cancer- study,
- Marijuana ingredient could be therapy for a deadly brain tumor, Augusta University finds,
- US Government finally admits that cannabis destroys cancer cells and protects healthy cells,

- 9 Science-Backed Benefits Of CBD Oil,
- 2021 was a record year for cannabis research. According to one analysis by the non-profit group NORML, more than 3,800 scientific papers were published on the topic of cannabis in the first eleven months of the year– a record high,
- Representatives from the National Institute on Drug Abuse (NIDA) and the Drug Enforcement Administration (DEA) recently voiced support for a White House proposal to expand researcher access to Schedule 1 drugs, such as cannabis and certain psychedelics,
- There are hundreds of efforts currently underway to standardize testing in the cannabis and hemp sectors. And while they're all welcome initiatives, there's one that carries a little more regulatory weight than the others: the National Institute of Science and Technology's (NIST's) Cannabis Quality Assurance Program (CannaQAP),
- Physicians See Patients Benefiting from Cannabis,
- FDA Approves IND Application for CBD Product Nantheia ATL5 (an investigational drug using cannabidiol (CBD) as an adjunctive treatment for opioid use disorder),
- Mississippi Researchers Awarded $1.37M to Study Cannabis Pain Relief Potential for HIV+ Patients
- Trial of Cannabidiol-derived EHP-101 for Relapsing MS Enrolling Soon.

WHERE DO WE GO FROM HERE?

The main goal for further research and development is to produce CBD products that continue to do a better job meeting the needs of patients who use them. Strict control of cannabis has severely limited scientific research into its many mysteries, which in turn, has had the ripple effect of a pretty significant knowledge gap regarding safe and effective medicinal uses. While the obvious outcomes scientists are looking for with the research are in line with using CBD effectively as medicine, the goals also include increased knowledge and understanding around how slight variations in the chemical make-up of different strains of cannabis offer different therapeutic properties, as well as the potential effects from cumulative exposure over time. Some of the areas where research is either underway or being considered include:

- Creating new and innovative products to better meet consumers' needs,
- Developing safer dosing methods for more precise ingestion of cannabis,
- Researching potential benefits for other health conditions yet to be explored.

The manufacturing process for CBD products includes four main stages: 1.) cultivation, 2.) extraction, 3.) processing and refining, and 4.) isolating valuable cannabinoids. Research is underway in all four stages.

1. CULTIVATION

The life cycle of cannabis plants includes several stages from choosing and germinating the seeds, to transplanting the seedlings, then monitoring them through the flowering stage, and finally harvesting when the time is right. Modifications in growing conditions have proven to successfully increase both the total yield and the cannabinoid content. Environmental conditions like the intensity and wavelength of light affect the chemical composition of the plants, and fertilization methods can impact the therapeutic properties of cannabis. Researchers are experimenting with growing temperatures, lighting, and irrigation, and about alternative pest control measures to prevent residual pesticides in the end products.

The ratio of compounds in each strain of plants is variable, so another area of research lies in developing CBD-rich strains. The goal is to create strains optimized for CBD content plus other therapeutic compounds like CBG, CBN, and certain specific terpenes. Recreational growers have developed numerous strains for high levels of THC, but so far, researchers have not been able to unlock the key to increasing the level of CBD in these genetically THC-rich strains. Doing so would be extremely beneficial since CBD can counteract some of the negative effects from taking too much THC. Researchers are exploring ways to best use certain strains with specific combinations of plant compounds to best help people living with different health conditions.

Auto-flowering seeds, which were created from older strains that are naturally rich in CBD are one way to get a CBD-rich seed. However, cannabis plants grown from seed could very easily express genetic features that might not represent the qualities the plants were bred for, so many growers prefer using clones. Growing and cultivation generate a lot of valuable data, so they offer a lot of possibilities for additional research.

Analyzing specific data helps prevent mold, fungus, and other issues related to environmental conditions. Monitoring plant growth and external conditions help predict the harvest date and the size of the yield, plus ideal watering schedules and other metrics, with remarkable precision. As the range of therapeutic uses for cannabis continues to expand, the need for a wider scope of research into all facets of the plant continues to increase, as well.

Another interesting area of research around cultivation includes using Artificial Intelligence (AI), which provides benefits to the CBD industry, including improvement of research processes. AI is used to monitor plant health and boost e-commerce personalization like targeted product search results and recommendations, and purchase-data analytics for online retailers.

Additionally, Smart Farming uses various technologies, including drones, so farmers can "see" their fields from the sky and respond to issues that are difficult to see from the ground. Benefits from smart farming include:

- Controlling growth areas. Near-infrared sensors on drones can provide growers with a view of the field and point out at-risk areas.
- Controlling fertilization and irrigation processes. Chemicals like pesticides and herbicides are virtually inevitable in large-scale farming, but drones help reduce the need for them by using GPS and ultrasonic echoing sensors to identify areas of concern. Then drones with sprayers are sent to treat weak areas. The same applies to the areas that need extra water and vital nutrients. Drones can reduce the need for manual labor and prevent exposure to chemicals.

2. EXTRACTION

The growth the hemp/CBD industry continues experiencing is outpacing the research needed to understand and explain the medicinal effects from the vast number of chemical compounds found primarily in the flowers of female cannabis plants. The discrepancy between the needs of the industry and the supporting research has resulted in confusing processes, products, and terms, so product development and methods of extraction have become important focal points. Thousands of chemical constituents have been identified in cannabis plants, all of which have different chemical properties requiring different conditions during the drying and extraction processes.

Cannabis manufacturers use different extraction methods that fall into three categories: rosin press extraction, short-path distillation and isolations, and finally, solvent-based extraction like we discussed in Chapter 1. Each of these extraction methods is used in the cannabis industry because each has different benefits.

Of all the compounds making up the chemistry of cannabis plants, terpenes are highly volatile compounds that can easily be lost in most common cannabinoid extraction processes. There is no ideal way to extract terpenes from organic sources, so researchers in the cannabis industry continue exploring new isolation methods. These delicate compounds require being handled with a little TLC.

One of the extraction methods currently being used is rosin presses, which extract cannabis resin containing dense concentrations of cannabinoids. Rosin technology is an innovative emerging technique that, unlike other resin extracting technologies, produces solvent-free cannabis concentrate without compromising quality. An effective rosin press combines a precisely determined amount of pressure with the lowest possible heat to minimize damage and maintain the original terpene profile of the plant.

Cannabis processors use Short-Path Distillation to separate cannabinoids from each other in order to purify and isolate them. Distillation is a method for separating compounds based on their unique physical properties like melting point, boiling point, and crystallization. One of the most common forms of distillation is by using boiling points. The result is a high-purity, superior quality concentrate that can be sold on its own or further processed into a variety of end products.

The major goals of research with extraction are to identify specific formulations and standard operating procedures to prepare and optimize Cannabis-based formulations. Considering that past studies were carried out using a variety of extraction processes and administered using differing dosages, the experiments were performed without proper control procedures. More research is needed to develop continuity and standards for extraction methods. Developing a green and sustainable cannabis extraction method is also being considered for future studies.

3. PROCESSING AND REFINING

Cannabis distillates and isolates are commonly used in vapes, edibles, and drinks, so these products are the main ingredients for pharmaceutical research. During this part of the process, the main goal is to mix the vegan product components without losing any of their important properties or using chemical additives and harmful compounds. The production process is highly technical: a raw cannabis extract is heated to different boiling points in order to extract various beneficial compounds, resulting in pure single-cannabinoid products. There are extraction systems that can create an isolate with up to 99.9% purity.

Chemically synthesized CBD is considered an attractive alternative for the pharmaceutical market because biosynthetic technology enhances consistency. Big Pharma prefers using synthetic or chemically synthesized CBD due to the element of control. Using synthetic compounds ensures high-purity and a consistent pharmaceutical product, which is not necessarily the case with naturally occurring, plant-based CBD products. While CBD can be easily extracted from the plant, other cannabinoids are not as accessible yet. Very little research has been done on the lesser-known cannabinoids, making it difficult to assess the potential demand for them as pharmaceutical ingredients. Using synthetic cannabinoids may be inevitable simply because of their consistent quality and affordable cost.

4. ISOLATION OF VALUABLE CANNABINOIDS

Although there is high demand for full-spectrum and broad-spectrum products in the consumer market, isolated cannabinoids have a bright future in multiple industries. From pharmaceutical-grade cannabinoid products to nutraceuticals, beauty and skincare to food and beverages, cannabinoid isolation has become critical to the industry.

Scientists have identified at least a hundred cannabinoids. While many of them probably have therapeutic effects, not every cannabis plant produces every cannabinoid, complicating the research processes. Years of strategic breeding would be necessary to create a stable supply chain of usable cannabis plants before significant research could be done with some of the rare compounds. However, researchers have identified a technique, known as biological synthesis, that involves engineering yeast, algae, or bacteria to produce compounds in a fermentation tank that will allow them to quickly generate cannabinoids without the time-line and complexity of growing cannabis plants.

This technology could fundamentally change the way cannabis products are sourced and consumed. It is particularly interesting because of the wide range of compounds with potential therapeutic qualities inherent in hemp plants and the difficulty involved with producing the compounds through either chemical synthesis or conventional plant breeding. Though questions remain about compounds isolated from cannabis plants, the rise of biosynthesis should accommodate the need for purified, consistent study drugs, which will speed up the processes of learning about each compound's potential benefits.

Cannabinoid biosynthesis companies are generally not interested in marijuana/THC because state marijuana markets are so tightly regulated. Rather, they are more interested in exploring the elusive compounds that are still holding tightly to their mysterious potential therapeutic benefits. Each cannabinoid seems to have a unique therapeutic effect, and they appear to have far-reaching influence over everything from blood sugar to migraines. As technology continues making the isolation process easier and more cost-effective, the market will continue to grow in order to accommodate more cannabinoid formulations with wider applications.

Another method for isolating cannabinoids that scientists and pharmaceutical companies are increasingly using is chromatography, a laboratory technique for isolating components from mixtures. A relatively simple process, flash chromatography is being used successfully by several processors in the hemp/cannabis industry to isolate specific cannabinoids. The industry's progress depends, to a large degree, on the ability to efficiently purify specific cannabinoids.

CLOSING THOUGHTS

To imagine the question of federal legalization for cannabis is no longer "If," but "When?" is very rewarding to a lot of people who have advocated for the medicinal value of cannabis for decades. However, unlike the vision many advocates have had over time, federal legalization probably won't be a blanket freedom to grow and use cannabis any old way you want. Rather, federal legalization is far more likely to be deeply entrenched in the patchwork web of various state regulations, and will absolutely be driven by the phenomenal amounts of money to be made by Big Pharma. Capitalism is a strong and mighty force! So, weighing in on federal legalization as a strict win for cannabis advocates isn't necessarily straight-forward.

But federal legalization is definitely on the horizon. And to that end, Big Pharma has made its power known in the medical cannabis arena. There is a certain irony to realize it is an insider path that has opened the door for legalization, to be sure. By providing a brief recap of a few of the various bills currently before Congress, we've made the point that legalization, whenever it occurs, will probably not look like the ideal many long-term marijuana advocates have envisioned.

In the meantime, research is proceeding at a faster pace than ever before. Restrictions are loosening, allowing for research down many paths that have previously been blocked. Scientists, doctors, and law-makers are all, finally, jumping on the band wagon, at least to a certain extent. We've seen the influence Big Pharma exerts over the government and the public, and we believe the only possible paths toward cannabis legalization will be focused on Big Pharma. The good news is that research is expanding at an extraordinary pace, and many people living with difficult-to-treat conditions are in line to benefit, even while Big Pharma leads the way.

After the Farm Bill was signed into law, many people in the hemp/CBD industry were worried the FDA would develop guidelines that might not represent the best interests of all the industry players. Not only has that not happened, but no guidelines at all have been developed, leaving the industry completely unregulated. Now the FDA has announced they don't plan to develop guidelines, and it looks like Congress is likely to be the arena to take on regulation for hemp/CBD, and the issue of guidelines will probably go hand-in-hand with legalization. For good or bad, or a little bit of both (?), Congress is likely to pick up where the FDA decided not to develop guidelines for the hemp/CBD industry.

BOLD EXPLORERS
BLAZING THE TRAIL

"I'M A DRUNK MINUS THE ALCOHOL!" though I am definitely not a dry-drunk! Black dots impair my vision, and I am challenged by both balance and mobility. My strength has gone the way of the wizard, to the point that I use an electric wheelchair.

My symptoms started in 1993, but then they really kicked into gear in 1999. I was working as a Certified Nursing Assistant (CNA) when I began experiencing numbness down the right side of my body; it got bad enough that I actually fell at work. One of the nurses I was working with insisted I needed to go to the hospital and have it checked out, but I wouldn't leave until my shift was over. In my heart, I just couldn't leave until my shift was finished.

When I got off at 9:00 P.M. I drove myself to a nearby hospital, despite the numbness, where they ran a bunch of tests, including an MRI, and I was diagnosed with Relapsing/Remitting Multiple Sclerosis. Relapsing/Remitting is just what it sounds like – you have a relapse, then go into remission for a while until you have another relapse. The relapses can vary in their strength and the amount of damage to your body. You go to bed one way and wake up another. It's crazy! I was only 27 years old.

Very quickly I got to the point that the entire right side of my body was numb, from my face and jawline all the way down to my foot and toes. My right hand and fingers began to curl, the right side of my face looked like I'd had a stroke. I couldn't sleep. Finally, I had to take a leave from work because performing my job had become impossible.

There's too much going on with this disease. One thing about MS is that most people's disease begins like mine did, relapsing and remitting, but it advances to what they call primary progressive, which is what I have now. It includes restless leg syndrome, though I've never been able to get a prescription to ease my restless legs. Some days my depression is so deep and dark that nothing helps with it. In the mornings, I have a runny nose. I have terrible headaches regularly. And I have pain all the way down my right side where the nerves are damaged. The nerves in my jowl are fried, so sometimes speaking and eating are difficult. I've lost close to 100 lbs. down from 219 to 125.

Several years ago, I decided to try Cannabis Medicine and I've gotten better results from taking CBD than from traditional meds. I take CBD in a tincture at night that helps me sleep and eases my restless legs. I have tried vaping the CBD oil and get a good result from that, as well. But I get the best result from smoking the flower, the same way people smoke marijuana. It works fast and offers me the best results. It helps with my headaches, and if I smoke just a little flower in the morning, it resolves my runny nose. I can now raise my right arm over my head, my right hand has uncurled, I can actually snap my fingers, and the pain is so much better! Even my depression is less horrible than it was before I started taking the CBD.

Chapter

9

THROUGHOUT THIS BOOK we've emphasized our belief that cannabis plants, and particularly CBD, as a product of cannabis plants, are medicinal. The United Nations and the World Health Organization agree; they are recommending CBD should not be scheduled under international drug conventions. The US government agrees, despite their collective refusal to publicly acknowledge this fact; they've legalized hemp-derived CBD products and removed them from Schedule 1 of the CSA. Furthermore, they've been holding a patent on several cannabinoids, including CBD, as neuroprotectants, contradicting their own definition of Schedule 1 drugs as having no accepted medical use. The American Medical Association agreed as far back as 1944; they're currently advocating for comprehensive, well-controlled studies to determine the role Cannabis Medicine should play in the treatment of diseases. More and more people in the US, including elected public officials, agree with us, demonstrated by the sheer number of people who are using CBD for medicinal purposes, coupled with the number of states with voter-approved, legal, medical marijuana programs. Big Pharma agrees with us; they're working diligently to create synthetic medicinal cannabinoids while simultaneously striving to limit access to natural cannabinoids because they compete in the market for their synthetic drugs.

In spite of all these entities agreeing that cannabis plants and CBD products are medicinal, we are still anxiously awaiting the day when a majority of traditional doctors and medical schools recognize Cannabis Medicine as a valid treatment option for patients, and begin teaching and learning Cannabis Medicine as a valid subject in accredited medical schools. As more and more doctors become knowledgeable about helping their patients understand and use Cannabis Medicine, there will always be two categories of people when it comes to cannabinoid-based medicine: those who trust Big Medicine, Big Pharma, and the FDA will remain a vital market for the cannabinoid medicines being developed and produced by Big Pharma, while those who are firm believers in natural healing and whole-plant medicines will remain in the CBD/medical marijuana market. Making sure both of these options are available in the future is critically important.

DISTINGUISHING BETWEEN CANNABIS MEDICINE AND ADULT RECREATIONAL MARIJUANA

Big Pharma has proven their ability and intent to provide options for those in the first category. For those in the second, we believe proceeding down a path of careful, vigilant adherence to a medical protocol is absolutely essential. In order to ensure continued access to a stable and expanding array of medicinal options of natural cannabinoid therapies, we believe the first step will be to carefully and rigorously distinguish the differences between Cannabis Medicine and the expanding market for adult recreational marijuana, especially once federal legalization occurs.

Recreational marijuana clearly has its place – it is more popular than ever, and is quickly being legalized in more and more states. But recreational marijuana and Cannabis Medicine are not the same thing, and continuously, relentlessly emphasizing the difference is paramount, and will continue to be. Remember, in the US, most CBD products are made from hemp, and hemp has absolutely no use as a recreational drug. That difference will be one of the most important elements for the ongoing success of an effective Cannabis Medicine market.

We believe one of the first steps in the direction of ensuring this difference would be to leave bud-tenders in charge of making recommendations for the adult recreational marijuana market, but to have pharmacists and/or other medical professionals in CBD stores and medical marijuana dispensaries. This idea is not new. When Connecticut passed its law legalizing medical marijuana in 2012, it became the first state to require pharmacists in dispensaries. The State of Louisiana licenses medical marijuana dispensaries as pharmacies. Minnesota and Arkansas both require pharmacists to be involved with dispensaries, and five other states require either a pharmacist or physician to be on staff. We believe this priority absolutely validates Cannabis Medicine as just that – a legitimate branch of medicine.

A CLEAR ROLE FOR PHARMACISTS

If embraced across the country, this practice will obviously require pharmacy schools to educate their students about Cannabis Medicine. Many of them are already doing so, and they're doing a great job! Pharmacy schools are offering programs focused on Cannabis Medicine not only for student pharmacists, but also for others, including those interested in regulatory and business purposes, and for improved patient care. A 2019 study from the University of Pittsburgh School of Pharmacy found 62% of US pharmacy schools surveyed had incorporated Medical Cannabis into their doctor of pharmacy programs, and another 23 percent planned to include similar courses in their programs within the next 12 months.[169] That's a much different outcome than those obtained from similar surveys of medical schools.

Many questions remain to be answered regarding the appropriate place for Cannabis Medicine in pharmaceutical treatment protocols. To begin answering those questions, the University of Florida College of Pharmacy is leading a statewide consortium studying health outcomes related to Cannabis Medicine. The consortium is tackling safety and effectiveness outcomes, plus challenges related to dosing, and analyzing how patients respond to smoking compared to other delivery methods. Another program at the University of the Sciences in Philadelphia offers a Medical Cannabis MBA program providing a combination of coursework in pharmaceutical, healthcare, and cannabis business. These are two examples of the visionary programs being undertaken through schools of pharmacy.

According to a 2020 article published in the *Journal of the American Pharmacists Association*:

> "… *pharmacists are in a unique position based on their accessibility, knowledge, and skills to guide product selection, dosing, and discuss drug interactions and adverse effects to educate patients on safe cannabis use. Pharmacists and pharmacy organizations should advocate for an integral role in the medical cannabis movement to ensure patient safety and evaluate cannabinoid pharmacology, pharmacokinetics, drug-drug interactions, safety, and efficacy through rigorous investigations.*"[170]

WHAT ABOUT DOCTORS?

A quick Google search shows a total of 19 medical schools in the US offering some form of education in Cannabis Medicine. Considering there are currently 155 accredited MD-granting institutions and 37 accredited DO-granting institutions in the United States, 19 seems like an awfully small number. We are cautiously optimistic for medical schools and medical doctors to begin recognizing the health benefits Cannabis Medicine offers patients, particularly in areas where traditional medicine and Cannabis Medicine are successfully working together. For doctors and medical schools to continue excluding Cannabis Medicine from their curriculums is a significant disservice to patients.

But all is not grim on this front. There are definitely medical doctors leading the way toward blending Cannabis Medicine with traditional medicine, even though they had to learn about Cannabis Medicine outside of traditional medical schools. Chapter 5 of this book is written by one. Some doctors are involved in a variety of efforts to share information with their colleagues about the patient-care opportunities Cannabis Medicine presents. We commend all of them!

WHAT DOES THE RESEARCH SHOW?

The ECS has become the most-studied retrograde signaling system in the human brain.[171] The results of these studies suggest manipulating ECS activity probably has therapeutic potential in almost all diseases affecting humans, and changes in ECS activity have been proven to demonstrate positive effects on an incredibly wide range of diseases. We've already discussed, back in Chapter 4, a few of the strategies for boosting endocannabinoids and how a combination of increasing endocannabinoids, combined with adding cannabinoids from cannabis plants, is one of the most effective ways to successfully manipulate the ECS. With this in mind, some producers of CBD products are beginning to add minor or "rare" cannabinoids to their products, in exact amounts and proportions, in order to offer consistent and reliable end-user experiences. Savvy customers are becoming very familiar with the effects they get from specific amounts of certain minor cannabinoids, in combination with specific potencies of CBD, and they are seeking not only specific ingredients, but specific ratios of these minor cannabinoids in their CBD products.

As consumers become more discerning about these types of products, several companies are now offering customers the option to create their own, customized cannabinoid blends in order to fine-tune their intake to meet their individual needs. This level of understanding about cannabinoids requires a tremendous amount of time and experimentation to figure out the exact "recipe" each body responds to best. Most people who have taken the time and energy to explore the range of possibilities this strategy represents in order to determine what works best for them have expressed how much they would appreciate having a knowledgeable doctor and/or pharmacist who could guide them through the process and eliminate, or at least minimize, the amount of trial and error they've undertaken.

WHERE DO WE GO FROM HERE?

As time goes on and medical research continues, doctors are realizing how many of the diseases affecting huge numbers of people actually give clues about their onset before symptoms begin, or as symptoms are just beginning. A series of blood tests is one of the first steps most doctors take when trying to figure out why a patient isn't feeling well, because most diseases have cellular indicators detectable in blood and/or urine samples. By the time a person is actually feeling crummy, a series of blood tests can check for things that might be out of balance and causing symptoms.

Additionally, people who are involved with the criminal justice system are generally subject to regular urinalyses designed to detect, among other things, the presence of THC, which used to be an indication the person was illegally smoking marijuana. Furthermore, some people whose jobs leave them subject to random drug tests must be prepared for not only urine and/or blood tests, but many are actually subject to having a tiny sample of their hair snipped and submitted to a laboratory to be tested for the presence of illegal drugs, including THC. However, since the passing of the 2018 Farm Bill, hemp products like CBD can legally have up to 0.3% THC, which is enough to show up in both blood and urine tests, so the presence of THC no longer necessarily means the person is using marijuana illegally. While this particular issue is clouded by the legal limit of THC being enough that it is detectable in blood and/or urine samples, the point is that modern medicine, as well as other institutions, already have systems in place that can measure the presence and levels of cannabinoids in the body.

Based on this fact alone, it is fairly obvious to see that blood tests will soon be available to determine the presence and level of specific cannabinoids, just like they can already determine the presence of THC, and cannabinoid levels found to be either too high or too low will prove to be accurate predictors for the onset of diseases associated with particular imbalances. With this in mind, it is a logical next step to anticipate responding to such imbalances with cannabinoid therapies. According to medical doctors who have been involved with this research, knowledge of the ECS will ultimately override the current medical system of managing and treating symptoms after someone has been diagnosed with a disease, and instead will create a system of disease prevention.

WILL MARKETING CBD CHANGE?

The CBD industry is already a multi-billion-dollar sector, and it is poised to continue growing. But valid CBD companies still have to navigate a maze of difficult hurdles, from accessing capital, to using standard payment processing, to being able to market their products through regular channels. A crucial development that will ease some of the burdens of these barriers is the FDA classifying CBD as a dietary supplement, whether by their own doing or by an act of Congress.

The ability to market CBD as a safe and effective substance is currently limited by the FDA's classification of it. Ultimately, the US Congress has the authority to address this issue, and there is legislation aiming to do just that, as we've presented earlier. Legislation will pave the way for the FDA to authorize marketing CBD as a dietary supplement, and this development will open up many marketing and distribution channels that remain either forbidden or restricted. Once companies are able to market CBD as a dietary supplement, it will flood mainstream retail.

Most huge companies have been hesitant to embrace CBD while it has been experiencing its initial growing pains, but once the regulatory landscape is cleared and stabilized, we believe many corporate giants will be looking to diversify their product lines with CBD. Companies like Procter & Gamble, Johnson & Johnson, Coca-Cola, and others will probably enter the market, and one of the ways they'll do so is by acquiring existing CBD market leaders. Additionally, public education about cannabinoids will become common as CBD continues going mainstream.

A POST-PANDEMIC CBD MARKET?

An interesting trend coming out of the COVID-19 pandemic is that people have become more mindful, and the collective consciousness is impacting things that previously seemed immune to this tendency, including the CBD market. Consumers expect more from brands, particularly with regard to social justice and environmental stewardship; and meeting consumer expectations has become an essential element for success in the CBD market. Millennials and Gen Z are driving the trend, holding brands to a higher social standard than ever before. These customers are interested in supporting companies that share their beliefs and values. According to the Porter-Novelli 2020 COVID-19 Tracker, 85% of Americans expect companies to help address racial inequality.[172] We believe the Cannabis Medicine market is in a position to make significant strides in easing some of the effects of the racist circumstances that have always been integral to both the War on Drugs and traditional healthcare systems.

Criminal justice reform and racial equity have become central issues in the national conversation around cannabis policy. As states pass cannabis reform laws or modify their existing laws, and Congress engages the issue in a more comprehensive way, efforts to reverse the *War on Drugs* and its effects have expanded significantly. As the Biden administration deals with a variety of crises at home and abroad, the coalition of voters who brought him to office -- liberals and progressives, people of color, women, young people, college-educated voters, and urban voters – are demanding the president do more on issues of race.

Connecting cannabis to issues of race and justice is not difficult. People of color are much more likely to be arrested for cannabis-related offenses despite usage rates being relatively equal. Cannabis policy in the US was designed, and has been implemented, to harm communities of color for generations, and given that intent, it has been a wildly successful policy endeavor. However, many Americans and people from both sides of the political divide see drug policy broadly and cannabis policy specifically for what it is, and that has led to a decades-long effort to step away from drug prohibition and criminalization and find a different policy path forward. In today's policy conversations, that path typically centers on cannabis reform.

Experts estimate the United States could gain $8 trillion by closing the racial equity gap, according to a report by the National Civic League.[173] Considering the hemp/CBD industry is strategically situated in the middle of the wellness space, the perception of aligned values matters more than ever. For many CBD businesses, this will mean focusing on the relatively untapped markets of African American and Hispanic customers. Cultural competence, particularly among the nation's largest brands, is likely to improve. Expect to see advertising focused on niche markets, and brand loyalty will shift toward the ones where consumers believe they are "seen." One of the first signs of brand dominance in a post-pandemic market will include strategic advertising campaigns specifically designed to appeal to Black and Hispanic consumers, coupled with Spanish language advertising, packaging, and support. Both Black and Hispanic consumers are likely to seek and support alternative products to help relieve pain, anxiety, sleep, and other conditions.[174]

The Hispanic market has grown in both size and influence over the last decade, so today, 62 million Hispanic consumers in the US have combined purchasing power of more than $1.5 trillion. In addition to representing a lucrative consumer audience, Hispanic consumers are more likely to rely on organic remedies, in part because of cultural norms and low access to traditional western medicine, coupled with a preference for alternative healthcare. Furthermore, the African American consumer market, with a consumer base of 48 million people who command $1.3 trillion in spending power, remains relatively untapped by CBD companies. Like Hispanic consumers, African Americans are less likely to seek treatment from traditional medical professionals, leaving a tremendous opportunity for forward-thinking CBD companies.

The Black and Hispanic markets are not likely to stay untapped much longer. Forward-thinking CBD brands are already making visible inroads. For example, the U.S. Hemp Roundtable, a coalition made up of dozens of leading companies and organizations committed to safe hemp/CBD products, recently announced their unanimous adoption of an equity and inclusion framework developed by the *Annie E. Casey Foundation*. This move, endorsed by industry leaders, signals a commitment to racial equity and inclusion in every link of the U.S. hemp industry.[175]

SUSTAINABILITY IN THE CANNABIS INDUSTRY

Environmental concerns are another hot-button for today's consumers, who are supporting sustainable farming by choosing products made using green practices. Hemp is in a position to become one of the most valuable crops grown in the contemporary world, and to do so in a green way. The National Cannabis Industry Association suggests that forward thinking, standard-setting bodies, self-regulatory organizations, and government regulators would be wise to create workable standards, with supporting resources, to set the cannabis industry apart as a leader in environmental sustainability. Strict regulations in the hemp market include numerous environmental protections, and more sustainable practices are being implemented regularly as the industry matures. Hemp/CBD businesses that incorporate environmentally sustainable practices will reduce negative impacts on the environment, while simultaneously increasing profit margins and saving their consumers money. These savings will be optimized if government partners collaborate with the industry to provide supporting resources, regulations, and policies.

The fast-growing and highly regulated hemp/CBD industry is in a position to become a leader on evolving agricultural challenges, especially by adopting environmentally sound business practices, proving to the larger agricultural sector that comprehensive environmental sustainability is achievable. The Hemp/CBD industry is poised to set the standards at minimizing environmental damage and the impact of climate change associated with traditional agriculture. For example, hemp minimizes radioactive and heavy metal contamination by literally absorbing these, and other harmful contaminants, from the soil. The cannabis industry will raise the bar with certain industrial farming practices like using pesticides and fertilizers, and replacing native vegetation with single-row, annually planted crops, which lead to unintended yet fully avoidable impacts to land use and soil health.[176]

Farmers love hemp as an eco-friendly crop. Growing hemp uses 50% less water than growing cotton, and it can also be used to make sustainable clothing. Hemp has valuable properties like removing toxins from the soil and cleansing it, making it suitable to sow other plants on a rotating basis. Perhaps the best benefit, though, is that hemp has long, deep roots that prevent soil erosion. Hemp helps the soil retain nutrients, plus it is resistant to pests, eliminating the need for toxic pesticides. Rather than needing conventional irrigation, farmers can grow hemp with harvested rainwater. Most importantly, hemp grows quickly in almost any climate, which means farmers can get multiple harvests throughout the year. Cultivating hemp requires lower land resources since the plants grow in closely packed clusters. And, since CBD extraction processes use carbon dioxide solvents, farming hemp minimizes the carbon footprint and helps reverse harmful effects through photosynthesis. Using CO_2 delivers CBD oil in its purest and safest form without toxic residues that pollute the rivers.

Hemp is essentially a zero-waste plant. The stalks, roots, flowers, and leaves, can be used to extract CBD oil. Fuel synthesized from the seeds has the potential to replace fossil-based petrol and gas. Hemp flour, tea, coffee, and milk are some of the consumables made by processing the seeds. The stalks are a rich source of fiber that can replace cotton, while other products are made from leaves and roots.

With increasing awareness about the ways traditional agriculture harms the environment, consumers are looking for cleaner and greener products. Because of the minimal need for chemicals, hemp farming is unlikely to cause long-term damage to the environment, so farmworkers, communities near the farmlands, and consumers all are able to avoid exposure to harmful chemicals. Also, most hemp products are packaged and delivered in recyclable and reusable containers, and microparticles don't make their way into waterways or pollute the oceans. Hemp products made with organic ingredients are entirely biodegradable.

CLOSING THOUGHTS

In spite of numerous entities, including the US government, agreeing with us that cannabis plants and CBD products are medicinal, we are still anxiously awaiting the day when a majority of traditional doctors and medical schools recognize Cannabis Medicine as a valid treatment option for patients, and begin teaching and learning Cannabis Medicine as a valid subject in accredited medical schools. As more and more doctors become knowledgeable about helping their patients understand and use Cannabis Medicine, there will always be two categories of people when it comes to cannabinoid-based medicine: those who trust Big Medicine, Big Pharma, and the FDA will remain a vital market for the cannabinoid medicines being developed and produced by Big Pharma, while those who are firm believers in natural healing and whole-plant medicines will remain in the CBD/medical marijuana market. Making sure both of these options are available in the future is critically important.

Big Pharma has proven their ability and intent to provide options for those in the first category. For those in the second, we believe proceeding down a path of careful, vigilant adherence to a medical protocol is absolutely essential. In order to ensure continued access to a stable and expanding array of medicinal options of natural cannabinoid therapies, we believe the first step will be to carefully and rigorously distinguish the differences between Cannabis Medicine and the expanding market for adult recreational marijuana, especially once federal legalization occurs. Recreational marijuana and Cannabis Medicine are not the same thing, and continuously, relentlessly emphasizing the difference is paramount, and will continue to be.

We believe one of the first steps in the direction of ensuring this difference would be to leave bud-tenders in charge of making recommendations for the adult recreational marijuana market, but to have pharmacists and/or other medical professionals in CBD stores and medical marijuana dispensaries. If embraced across the country, this practice will obviously require pharmacy schools to educate their students about Cannabis Medicine. We are cautiously optimistic for medical schools and medical doctors to begin recognizing the health benefits Cannabis Medicine offers patients, particularly in areas where traditional medicine and Cannabis Medicine are successfully working together. For doctors and medical schools to continue excluding Cannabis Medicine from their curriculums is a significant disservice to patients.

The ECS has become the most-studied retrograde signaling system in the human brain. The results of these studies suggest manipulating ECS activity probably has therapeutic potential in almost all diseases affecting humans, and changes in ECS activity have been proven to demonstrate positive effects on an incredibly wide range of diseases. Some producers of CBD products are beginning to add minor or "rare" cannabinoids to their products, in exact amounts and proportions, in order to offer consistent and reliable end-user experiences. Savvy customers are becoming very familiar with the effects they get from specific amounts of certain minor cannabinoids, in combination with specific potencies of CBD, and they are seeking not only specific ingredients, but specific amounts and ratios of these minor cannabinoids in their CBD products. Most people who have taken the time and energy to explore the range of possibilities this strategy represents in order to determine what works best for them have expressed how much they would appreciate having a knowledgeable doctor and/or pharmacist who could guide them through the process and eliminate, or at least minimize, the amount of trial and error they've undertaken.

Blood tests will soon be available to determine the presence and level of specific cannabinoids, just like they can already determine the presence of THC. If certain cannabinoid levels are found to be either too high or too low, they will be accurate predictors for the onset of diseases associated with particular imbalances. It is a logical next step to anticipate responding to such imbalances with cannabinoid therapies.

The ability to market CBD as a safe and effective substance is currently limited by the FDA's classification of it. Once companies are able to market CBD as a dietary supplement, it will flood mainstream retail. Huge companies will probably enter the market, and one of the ways they'll do so is to purchase existing CBD market leaders.

An interesting trend coming out of the COVID-19 pandemic is that many people have become more mindful, and the collective consciousness is impacting things that previously seemed immune to this tendency, including the CBD market. Consumers expect more from brands, particularly with regard to social justice and the climate, and meeting consumer expectations has become an essential element for success in the CBD market. We believe the Cannabis Medicine market is in a position to make significant strides in easing some of the effects of the racist circumstances that have always been integral to both the War on Drugs and the traditional healthcare systems.

Environmental concerns are another hot-button for today's consumers, who are supporting sustainable farming by choosing products created with green practices. Hemp is positioned to become one of the most valuable crops in the world, and to do so in a green way. With increasing awareness about the ways traditional agriculture is harmful to the environment, consumers are looking for cleaner and greener options, and hemp-derived CBD products fit the bill.

EPILOGUE

THIS BOOK CAME ABOUT BECAUSE of my personal interest in learning as much as I could about CBD. When I realized how difficult it was to find viable information, I wanted to make it easier to access for others who wanted the same thing – legitimate information about CBD.

I began taking CBD shortly after I started my research, feeling like it was definitely something I wanted to try. And the more I learned, the more I believed it would be an oversight for me not to take it. Like most of the other people whose testimonials are included in the book, my doctor did not discourage me from trying it, though he was not helpful, either. I've been lucky because I met Eric, and plenty of other people in the industry who are knowledgeable and helpful.

Most of my MS symptoms have eased since I started taking CBD. My bone density has improved, my muscle spasms have eased, my brain fog is considerably better. My depression and anxiety have eased, and my insomnia is better. Unfortunately, MS is a weird disease, so it's impossible to say with certainty that these results are because of the CBD. Truthfully, maybe they would have eased anyway. That possibility is extremely unlikely, but who knows?

I have an experience with CBD that I hope will inspire others who might not be seeing the results they were hoping for. Like I said, I've been taking CBD for three years. I started out taking capsules, but at some point, shifted to a tincture. I've been taking a tincture that offers a blend of CBD with a couple other cannabinoids, and though I've generally gotten a great response from them, I had one lingering symptom that seemed not to respond to the CBD at all. Chronic pain.

I get excruciating pain on the right side of my neck, through my right shoulder, and down into my right arm. I've been dealing with this agonizing pain for well over a decade. When doctors have asked me that inevitable question of how much pain I have on a scale of 1 to 10, I wanted to scream, "On a scale of 1 to 10, it's a 500!!!!!"

But here's the interesting thing. There's nothing wrong with my neck, shoulder, or upper arm. The damaged tissue is in my spinal cord in my neck. I have MS lesions in my neck. So, I have been faced with the illusive question of how to treat pain that hurts where there isn't any damaged tissue? After trying everything we could think of, I finally started taking opioids for pain relief. I've been taking prescription opioids for years and years, which creates a lot of difficult issues with prescriptions and pharmacies and insurance, etc., not to mention side effects. Though the opioids help with my pain management, I've tried many times to get off of them, but without success because the pain is just too intense.

Then out of the blue, one day I tried a topical salve blended with the same mixture I've been taking as a tincture. I mention this to emphasize that my body was accustomed to this blend – I'd been taking it for about a year. One evening I rubbed the salve on my neck, shoulder, and upper arm, and was absolutely shocked to realize I was pain-free! I didn't think I'd ever be able to say that. It seems like a million years ago since I didn't have the pain.

I've now been using the salve for a couple months, and I'm taking a lower dose of prescription pain medication than I have in a decade. I'm weaning off of them slowly, as my body has become dependent. I continue taking the tincture, plus I use the salve twice daily, and I am awfully close to living pain free.

So, if you haven't yet found a CBD product and/or delivery method that works for you, keep trying. Continue experimenting with different methods of taking the CBD, with different brands, different combinations of cannabinoids, and different delivery methods. On some level it seems kind of obvious that I should have tried the salve sooner, but I doubted treating the neck/shoulder/arm would work because the damage is actually in my neck. But believe me when I say I am thrilled to use it daily for the rest of my life!

To everyone who reads this book, I truly wish you the best on your wellness journey! For some people, health is an easier journey than for others, but each of us faces our unique circumstances. Don't give up -- try everything! Keep trying until you find something that works. I hope you've learned enough about CBD to decide for yourself whether you want to give it a try.

This book came about because of a shared frustration over how difficult it is, or has been, to find valid information about CBD. After conducting hours and hours and hours of research about CBD and Cannabis Medicine, what we really care about telling you is that Catherine can truly say her MS symptoms have improved with CBD in ways that seem impossible with traditional western medicine.

We've included testimonials from several other people who agree that CBD has offered them improved health outcomes that were otherwise not available to them, including hope for a healthy future. That's what this book is really about -- Hope. Hope for effective treatments for so many diseases and conditions that remain elusive to modern medicine. Hope for improved health for so many people living with diseases that are not understood. Hope for younger generations, that they might not have to experience many of the health challenges facing older generations.

For anyone, everyone, out in the world who is struggling with mysterious symptoms, or has received a diagnosis that feels like a death sentence, or is simply not feeling as good as you wish you could, please read this book. Read the information and the testimonials. Check our resources. Don't give up! People living with all kinds of health conditions that are difficult to treat, or that don't respond well to traditional medicines, or who have mysterious symptoms that somehow haven't fit into a diagnosis, have been able to make surprising strides with CBD. Though it is definitely not a cure-all, CBD has helped multitudes of people living with multitudes of health challenges, and you could be among them.

While most people have heard a little something-something about CBD, few really understand what it is, what it is not, why it works the way it does, and how to get started on a CBD therapy. Not many doctors are prepared to provide answers for their patients seeking information about how CBD might help them with their personal health challenges. This fact alone leaves plenty of people wondering why doctors are not more enthusiastic about CBD, and many feel concerned about trying it since their doctors are not supportive. Complicating the picture, there are literally thousands of webpages with information about CBD, but if you start reading them carefully, you quickly realize much of the information is contradictory. This leaves people unsure what to believe or where to turn when they still have questions.

We've tried to provide the information we feel is important for people to know and understand about CBD, but there is still so much more information out in the world! For what it's worth, we estimate that only about 25% of the material we wrote with the intention of including in this book actually ended up here. There are a number of reasons why, and we make this statement here just to let you know that we've barely scratched the surface of information about Cannabis Medicine in general, and CBD in particular.

A variety of themes are woven throughout the book, including the lengthy history of Cannabis Medicine. People have been using cannabis plants as medicine for thousands of years. Despite this fact, there remains a dark stigma about the merits of CBD and other forms of Cannabis Medicine among some very important groups of people that carry a lot of weight, including most medical professionals and the federal government. We've tried to explain some of the reasons for these circumstances, and to discuss what the future appears to hold. We encourage all medical professionals to learn as much as possible about Cannabis Medicine, the ECS, and CBD in order to help guide their patients in the direction of remedies that are otherwise not available. We know patients are interested in feeling better, and we know a lot of people who started feeling a whole lot better with CBD therapies than they did without them. All of these people, plus many others, would sure appreciate having medical professionals able to help guide them through the process of getting started and continuing down the path of using CBD. With regard to the federal government, we are definitely not conspiracy theorists, but there sure seems to be a certain amount of the right hand and the left hand not coordinating their actions to efficiently juggle the issues of Cannabis Medicine. As we've stated throughout the book, we have absolutely no interest in painting a negative picture of the federal government or any of its agencies or departments. We are only trying to clear the muck of information about CBD, and the government seems to be entrenched in much of it.

However, the FDA has, for the first time ever, approved a cannabinoid-based medication. Epidiolex is officially approved as a treatment for specific forms of pediatric epilepsy. With this approval, many people are hopeful for approvals of additional cannabinoid-based medications in the future. And while some people see this as an indicator that federal legalization is not too far down the road, another reason some people believe legalization might finally be poised to happen is that the US federal government has been holding a patent on several cannabinoids, including CBD, as neuroprotectants. With this patent, the US Department of Health and

Human Services has confirmed what many people have been advocating for decades, that cannabinoid medicine is real, and it offers wellness options that are otherwise not available.

The question of federal marijuana legalization is widely believed to be a question of "When?" rather than "If?" There are several bills before Congress that include some form of legalization. On the surface, this possibility seems like a win for people who have been advocating for legalization for years. However, when federal legalization does occur, it will probably not include the freedom to plant and use cannabis whenever and however anybody wants. Rather, it is much more likely to reflect the asymmetry of the state-level medical marijuana laws and the same kinds of strict government oversight that hemp is subject to. But the pendulum is in full swing.

Living a healthy lifestyle is not necessarily easy. These are difficult times for everyone. The pandemic and its economic fall-out have affected everyone. People are feeling pressure and stress from all directions, which takes a toll on everyone's health sooner or later. For many people, the incidence of mental health challenges and physical health challenges seem to play out as some crazy kind of chicken-and-egg scenario. Some people begin feeling mental health challenges after a certain amount of time dealing with physical health challenges. For others, the exact opposite occurs. But either way, people are seeking help.

We believe CBD can offer many the help they seek. Wherever you are on your personal wellness journey, we believe information is power. Hopefully, you have found enough information here to leave you feeling powerful about deciding whether or not CBD is for you.

ACKNOWLEDGMENTS

SO MANY PEOPLE HAVE CONTRIBUTED to the making of this book! How can we ever name everyone?

Special thanks to Dr. Sharon Montes, not only for your contribution to the book, but for your kindness and generosity of both time and energy, for your insights, knowledge, and professionalism at every step. To the amazing people whose stories are included as *Bold Explorers Blazing the Trail:* Shamay, Robbie, Robert, Sherri, Kelli, Andra, Eileen, and John Doe – you know who you are. We are grateful for the privilege of sharing your stories and your adventurous spirits with all of our readers. To Ryan Smith for your help and insights, your humor, and especially for keeping us (especially Catherine) calm when things seemed like they were either moving too fast or not fast enough. Thanks to the team at Botanacor, and Ashton Hendricks, for your help with the COA. Thanks to Pauline Verbest for your wonderful illustrations and graphics, and to Irene Neybert for your insights and suggestions. Thanks to Dr. Rege Hastings for your guidance about the science section. Thank you to the members of Catherine's weekly writers' group – Scott, Marcia, Elsa, Layne, Marco, John, Doc -- for your thoughtful recommendations and moral support along the path. Thanks to all who gave us your time and strategic feedback – especially Justin Durbin, Caleb Shaver, and Ryan Groves. And thanks to all of our friends and families who believed in us, even when you wondered what in the world we were trying to do by writing a book about CBD oil. With the help from all of you, and countless others, WE DID IT!!

ENDNOTES

1   2019. Hempbizjournal.com. 2019

2   "IAPT - International Association for Plant Taxonomy." n.d. IAPT. https://www.iapt-global.org.

3   Campbell, Todd. 2019. "Hemp vs. Marijuana: What's the Difference?"

4   The Motley Fool. February 9, 2019. https://www.fool.com/investing/2019/02/09/hemp-vs-marijuana-whats-the-difference.aspx.

5   Wholisticmatters.com. 2022. https://wholisticmatters.com/wp-content/uploads/2019/09/Cannabis-Overview-Cover-Image.png.

6   "Race and the Drug War." n.d. Drug Policy Alliance. https://www.drugpolicy.org/issues/race-and-drug-war.

7   LoBianco, Tom. 2016. "Report: Nixon's War on Drugs Targeted Black People." CNN. March 24, 2016. https://www.cnn.com/2016/03/23/politics/john-ehrlichman-richard-nixon-drug-war-blacks-hippie/index.html.

8   Milutin. 2019. "World Health Organization Recommends Reclassifying Marijuana under International Treaties." Drug Policy Network SEE. February 11, 2019. https://dpnsee.org/2019/02/11/world-health-organization-recommends-reclassifying-marijuana-under-international-treaties/

9   "Why Does Cannabis Potency Matter?" n.d. United Nations: Office on Drugs and Crime. https://www.unodc.org/unodc/en/frontpage/2009/June/why-does-cannabis-potency-matter.html

10   "Report: Majority of Commercially Available CBD Products 'Contaminated' with Heavy Metals." n.d. NORML.

11   Paul, Alan. 2019. "How Is CBD Oil Made - the Process Explained." Urbul. March 28, 2019. https://www.urbul.com/blog/how-is-cbd-oil-made.

12   "Nuance Communications, Inc." 2013. https://www.justice.gov/iso/opa/resour ces/3052013829132756857467.pdf

13   Office of the Commissioner. 2019. "FDA Regulation of Cannabis and Cannabis-Derived Products: Q&A." U.S. Food and Drug Administration. 2019. https://www.fda.gov/news-events/public-health-focus/ fda-regulation-cannabis-and-cannabis-derived-products-including-cannabidiol-cbd.

14   Surprenant, Zac. 2021. "Label Requirements for CBD and Cannabis Products | Bennett." BPKC. July 26, 2021. https://bpkc.com/ label-requirements-for-cbd-and-cannabis-products/.

15   "Congress Moves to End Nixon's Drug War on 50th Anniversary." 2021. The Leaf Online. June 17, 2021. http://theleafonline.com/c/other-drugs/2021/06/ congress-renews-effort-to-end-nixons-drug-war-on-50th-anniversary/.

16   Jaeger, Kyle. 2021. "First-Ever Congressional Bill to Decriminalize All Drugs Announced ahead of Nixon Drug War Anniversary." Marijuana Moment. June 15, 2021. https://www.marijuanamoment.net/first-ever-congressional-bill-to-decriminal- ize-all-drugs-introduced-ahead-of-nixon-drug-war-anniversary/.

17   News, Marijuana. 2021. "DEA Is Allowing More Research of Cannabis, but Some Silly Roadblocks Remain." 420 Intel. June 11, 2021. http://420intel.com/articles/2021/06/11/ dea-allowing-more-research-cannabis-some-silly-roadblocks-remain.

18   Jaeger, Kyle. 2021. "Congressional Bill to Federally Legalize Marijuana Filed by Republican Lawmakers." Marijuana Moment. May 12, 2021. https://www.marijuanamoment.net/ congressional-bill-to-federally-legalize-marijuana-filed-by-republican-lawmakers/.

19   Downing, Nicholas S., Nilay D. Shah, Jenerius A. Aminawung, Alison M. Pease, Jean-David Zeitoun, Harlan M. Krumholz, and Joseph S. Ross. 2017. "Postmarket Safety Events among Novel Therapeutics Approved by the US Food and Drug Administration between 2001 and 2010." *JAMA* 317 (18): 1854. https://doi. org/10.1001/jama.2017.5150

20   Ewing, Laura E., Charles M. Skinner, Charles M. Quick, Stefanie Kennon-McGill, Mitchell R. McGill, Larry A. Walker, Mahmoud A. ElSohly, Bill J. Gurley, and Igor Koturbash. 2019. "Hepatotoxicity of a Cannabidiol-Rich Cannabis Extract in the Mouse Model." *Molecules* 24 (9): 1694. https://doi.org/10.3390/molecules24091694

21   "Dronabinol Uses, Side Effects & Warnings." n.d. Drugs.com. https://www.drugs.com/ mtm/dronabinol.html.

22   "Nabilone." Drugs.com. Drugs.com. 2019. https://www.drugs.com/mtm/nabilone. html.

23   Office of the Commissioner. 2019. "FDA Regulation of Cannabis and Cannabis-Derived Products: Q&A." U.S. Food and Drug Administration. 2019. https://www.fda.gov/news-events/public-health-focus/ fda-regulation-cannabis-and-cannabis-derived-products-including-cannabidiol-cbd.

24   U.S. Department of Health and Human Services. 2016. "About HHS." HHS.gov. March 18, 2016.

25   "US6630507B1 - Cannabinoids as Antioxidants and Neuroprotectants - Google Patents." 1999. Google.com. April 21, 1999. https://patents.google.com/patent/ US6630507B1/en.

26   "US6630507B1 - Cannabinoids as Antioxidants and Neuroprotectants - Google Patents." 1999. Google.com. April 21, 1999. https://patents.google.com/patent/ US6630507B1/en.

27   "U.S. Domestic Hemp Production Program | Agricultural Marketing Service." n.d.

28   Www.ams.usda.gov. https://www.ams.usda.gov/rules-regulations/hemp.

29   "Electronic Code of Federal Regulations (ECFR)." n.d. Electronic Code of Federal Regulations (ECFR). https://www.ecfr.gov/.https://www.ecfr.gov/current/title-7/ subtitle-B/chapter-IX/part-990/subpart-C

30   "The USDA Rules in Detail: Testing Requirements." 2019. The Pipeline Cannabis Law Advisor. November 7, 2019.

31   "Farm Bill." n.d. Www.usda.gov. https://www.usda.gov/farmbill.

32   Hudak, John. 2018. "The Farm Bill, Hemp Legalization and the Status of CBD: An Explainer." Brookings. Brookings. December 14, 2018. https://www.brookings.edu/ blog/fixgov/2018/12/14/the-farm-bill-hemp-and-cbd-explainer/.

33   Nih.gov. 2017. https://ods.od.nih.gov/About/DSHEA_Wording.aspx.

34   2017. Nih.gov. 2017. https://ods.od.nih.gov/About/DSHEA_Wording.aspx.https:// ods.od.nih.gov/About/DSHEA_Wording.aspx

35   Nettlemere. n.d. "Medicines Derived from Plants." YouMeMindBody. https://youme- mindbody.com/health-care-industry/Medicines-Derived-from-Plants.

36   Vickers, A. 2001. "Herbal Medicine." *Western Journal of Medicine* 175 (2): 125–28. https://doi.org/10.1136/ewjm.175.2.125.

37   Girard, Lauren, and Sunita Vohra. 2011. "Ethics of Using Herbal Medicine as Primary or Adjunct Treatment and Issues of Drug-Herb Interaction." Nih.gov. CRC Press/ Taylor & Francis. 2011. https://www.ncbi.nlm.nih.gov/books/NBK92754/.

38   Lemonnier, Nathanaël, Guang-Biao Zhou, Bhavana Prasher, Mitali Mukerji, Zhu Chen, Samir K. Brahmachari, Denis Noble, Charles Auffray, and Michael Sagner. 2017. "Traditional Knowledge-Based Medicine." *Progress in Preventive Medicine* 2 (7): e0011. https://doi.org/10.1097/pp9.0000000000000011.

39   "WHO GLOBAL REPORT on TRADITIONAL and COMPLEMENTARY MEDICINE 2019." n.d. https://www.who.int/traditional-complementary-integrative-medicine/WhoGlobalReportOnTraditionalAndComplementaryMedicine2019.pdf.

40   "The Emergence and Evolution of Botanicals in Cosmetics." 2019. *Sensient Beauty.* July 24, 2019. https://www.sensient-cosmetics.com/the-emergence-and-evolution-of-botanicals-in-cosmetics/#:~:text=%E2%80%9CBetween%201990%20and%201997%2C%20the.

41   Vickers, A. 2001. "Herbal Medicine." *Western Journal of Medicine* 175 (2): 125–28. https://doi.org/10.1136/ewjm.175.2.125.

42   Russo, Ethan B. 2008. "Cannabinoids in the Management of Difficult to Treat Pain." *Therapeutics and Clinical Risk Management* 4 (1): 245–59. https://www.ncbi.nlm.nih.gov/pmc/articles/PMC2503660/.

43   Russo, Ethan B. 2016. "Current Therapeutic Cannabis Controversies and Clinical Trial Design Issues." *Frontiers in Pharmacology* 7 (September). https://doi.org/10.3389/fphar.2016.00309.

44   Pamplona, Fabricio A., Lorenzo Rolim da Silva, and Ana Carolina Coan. 2018. "Potential Clinical Benefits of CBD-Rich Cannabis Extracts over Purified CBD in Treatment-Resistant Epilepsy: Observational Data Meta-Analysis." *Frontiers in Neurology* 9 (September). https://doi.org/10.3389/fneur.2018.00759.

45   Flavonoids. 2014. "Flavonoids." Linus Pauling Institute. April 28, 2014. https://lpi.oregonstate.edu/mic/dietary-factors/phytochemicals/flavonoids.

46   "Flavones - an Overview | ScienceDirect Topics." n.d. Www.sciencedirect.com. Accessed April 27, 2022. https://www.sciencedirect.com/topics/agricultural-and-biological-sciences/flavones.

47   Khoo, Hock Eng, Azrina Azlan, Sou Teng Tang, and See Meng Lim. 2017. "Anthocyanidins and Anthocyanins: Colored Pigments as Food, Pharmaceutical Ingredients, and the Potential Health Benefits." *Food & Nutrition Research* 61 (1): 1361779. https://doi.org/10.1080/16546628.2017.1361779.

48   "Flavanones - an Overview | ScienceDirect Topics." n.d. Www.sciencedirect.com. https://www.sciencedirect.com/topics/agricultural-and-biological-sciences/flavanones.

49   "Isoflavones - an Overview | ScienceDirect Topics." n.d. Www.sciencedirect.com. https://www.sciencedirect.com/topics/agricultural-and-biological-sciences/isoflavones.

50   PubChem. n.d. "Flavanone." Pubchem.ncbi.nlm.nih.gov. https://pubchem.ncbi.nlm.nih.gov/compound/flavanone?msclkid=99a65fc8a79f11ec86cbbc7d23807e3d.

51   Osakabe, Naomi. 2013. "Flavan 3-Ols Improve Metabolic Syndrome Risk Factors: Evidence and Mechanisms." *Journal of Clinical Biochemistry and Nutrition* 52 (3): 186–92. https://doi.org/10.3164/jcbn.12-130.

52   Rodríguez-García, Carmen, Cristina Sánchez-Quesada, and José J. Gaforio. 2019. "Dietary Flavonoids as Cancer Chemopreventive Agents: An Updated Review of Human Studies." *Antioxidants* 8 (5): 137. https://doi.org/10.3390/antiox8050137

53   Ullah, Asad, Sidra Munir, Syed Lal Badshah, Noreen Khan, Lubna Ghani, Benjamin Gabriel Poulson, Abdul-Hamid Emwas, and Mariusz Jaremko. 2020. "Important Flavonoids and Their Role as a Therapeutic Agent." *Molecules* 25 (22): 5243. https://doi.org/10.3390/molecules25225243.

54   "Simple Dietary Changes May Reduce Cancer Risk, Increase Lifespan." 2019. Www. medicalnewstoday.com. August 16, 2019. https://www.medicalnewstoday.com/articles/326042#500-mg-each-day.

55   Sandoval, Viviana, Hèctor Sanz-Lamora, Giselle Arias, Pedro F. Marrero, Diego Haro, and Joana Relat. 2020. "Metabolic Impact of Flavonoids Consumption in Obesity: From Central to Peripheral." *Nutrients* 12 (8): 2393. https://doi.org/10.3390/nu12082393.

56   "Home-Center for Medical Weight Loss." 2022. Centerformedicalweightloss. com. 2022. https://www.centerformedicalweightloss.com/fitnessexerice_article. aspx?url=Eat%20Your%20Flavonoids.

57   "George Mateljan, Founder." n.d. Whfoods.com. http://www.whfoods.com/genpage. php?tname=biosketch&dbid=3.

58   Cordain, Loren, S Boyd Eaton, Anthony Sebastian, Neil Mann, Staffan Lindeberg, Bruce A Watkins, James H O'Keefe, and Janette Brand-Miller. 2005. "Origins and Evolution of the Western Diet: Health Implications for the 21st Century." *The American Journal of Clinical Nutrition* 81 (2): 341–54. https://doi.org/10.1093/ajcn.81.2.341.

59   "Flavonoids > Defeat Diabetes Foundation." n.d. Defeat Diabetes Foundation. https:// defeatdiabetes.org/resources/healthful-eating/nutrients/flavonoids/.

60   Li, Z., S. M. Henning, Y. Zhang, N. Rahnama, A. Zerlin, G. Thames, C. H. Tseng, and D. Heber. 2013. "Decrease of Postprandial Endothelial Dysfunction by Spice Mix Added to High-Fat Hamburger Meat in Men with Type 2 Diabetes Mellitus." *Diabetic Medicine: A Journal of the British Diabetic Association* 30 (5): 590–95. https://doi.org/10.1111/dme.12120.

61   "Linus Pauling Institute." n.d. Linus Pauling Institute. https://lpi.oregonstate.edu/.

62   Peterson, J, P Lagiou, E Samoli, A Lagiou, K Katsouyanni, C La Vecchia, J Dwyer, and D Trichopoulos. 2003. "Flavonoid Intake and Breast Cancer Risk: A Case–Control Study in Greece." *British Journal of Cancer* 89 (7): 1255–59. https://doi.org/10.1038/sj.bjc.6601271.

63   Chen, Allen Y., and Yi Charlie Chen. 2013. "A Review of the Dietary Flavonoid, Kaempferol on Human Health and Cancer Chemoprevention." *Food Chemistry* 138 (4): 2099–2107. https://doi.org/10.1016/j.foodchem.2012.11.139.

64 Shishtar, Esra, Gail T. Rogers, Jeffrey B. Blumberg, Rhoda Au, and Paul F. Jacques. 2020. "Long-Term Dietary Flavonoid Intake and Risk of Alzheimer Disease and Related Dementias in the Framingham Offspring Cohort." *The American Journal of Clinical Nutrition* 112 (2): 343–53. https://doi.org/10.1093/ajcn/nqaa079.

65 Publishing, Harvard Health. 2021. "Foods Linked to Better Brainpower." Harvard Health. March 6, 2021. https://www.health.harvard.edu/healthbeat/foods-linked-to-better-brainpower.

66 "Validate User." n.d. Academic.oup.com. https://academic.oup.com/aje/article/165/12/1364/125579.

67 Ferraz, Carvalho, Manchope, Artero, Rasquel-Oliveira, Fattori, Casagrande, and Verri. 2020. "Therapeutic Potential of Flavonoids in Pain and Inflammation: Mechanisms of Action, Pre-Clinical and Clinical Data, and Pharmaceutical Development." *Molecules* 25 (3): 762. https://doi.org/10.3390/molecules25030762.

68 Ferraz, Carvalho, Manchope, Artero, Rasquel-Oliveira, Fattori, Casagrande, and Verri. 2020. "Therapeutic Potential of Flavonoids in Pain and Inflammation: Mechanisms of Action, Pre-Clinical and Clinical Data, and Pharmaceutical Development." *Molecules* 25 (3): 762. https://doi.org/10.3390/molecules25030762.

69 Zakaryan, Hovakim, Erik Arabyan, Adrian Oo, and Keivan Zandi. 2017. "Flavonoids: Promising Natural Compounds against Viral Infections." *Archives of Virology* 162 (9): 2539–51. https://doi.org/10.1007/s00705-017-3417-y.

70 "Linus Pauling Institute." n.d. Linus Pauling Institute. https://lpi.oregonstate.edu/.

71 "What Are Cannabis Flavonoids and Why Do They Matter?" 2020. *The Higher Path Collective.* January 2, 2020. https://www.thehigherpath.com/cannabis-flavonoids/.

72 Russo, Ethan B. 2008. "Cannabinoids in the Management of Difficult to Treat Pain." *Therapeutics and Clinical Risk Management* 4 (1): 245–59. https://www.ncbi.nlm.nih.gov/pmc/articles/PMC2503660/.

73 Moreau, Michele, Udoka Ibeh, Kaylie Decosmo, Noella Bih, Sayeda Yasmin-Karim, Ngeh Toyang, Henry Lowe, and Wilfred Ngwa. 2019. "Flavonoid Derivative of Cannabis Demonstrates Therapeutic Potential in Preclinical Models of Metastatic Pancreatic Cancer." *Frontiers in Oncology* 9 (July). https://doi.org/10.3389/fonc.2019.00660.

74 Hess, Peter. n.d. "Pain-Killing Compound 30 Times Stronger than Aspirin Revealed in Cannabis." *Inverse.* https://www.inverse.com/article/58027-cannflavins-a-and-b-in-cannabis-anti-inflammatory.

75 Radwan, Mohamed M., Mahmoud A. ElSohly, Desmond Slade, Safwat A. Ahmed, Lisa Wilson, Abir T. El-Alfy, Ikhlas A. Khan, and Samir A. Ross. 2008. "Non-Cannabinoid Constituents from a High Potency Cannabis Sativa Variety." *Phytochemistry* 69 (14): 2627–33. https://doi.org/10.1016/j.phytochem.2008.07.010.

76 Li, Yao, Jiaying Yao, Chunyan Han, Jiaxin Yang, Maria Chaudhry, Shengnan Wang, Hongnan Liu, and Yulong Yin. 2016. "Quercetin, Inflammation and Immunity." *Nutrients* 8 (3): 167. https://doi.org/10.3390/nu8030167.

77 "Luteolin - an Overview | ScienceDirect Topics." n.d. Www.sciencedirect.com. Accessed April 27, 2022. https://www.sciencedirect.com/topics/neuroscience/luteolin.

78 Alam, M. Ashraful, Nusrat Subhan, M. Mahbubur Rahman, Shaikh J. Uddin, Hasan M. Reza, and Satyajit D. Sarker. 2014. "Effect of Citrus Flavonoids, Naringin and Naringenin, on Metabolic Syndrome and Their Mechanisms of Action." *Advances in Nutrition* 5 (4): 404–17. https://doi.org/10.3945/an.113.005603.

79 Zhang, Rui, In Kyung Lee, Mei Jing Piao, Ki Cheon Kim, Areum Daseul Kim, Hye Sun Kim, Sungwook Chae, Hee Sun Kim, and Jin Won Hyun. 2011. "Butin (7,3⊠,4⊠-Trihydroxydihydroflavone) Reduces Oxidative Stress-Induced Cell Death via Inhibition of the Mitochondria-Dependent Apoptotic Pathway." *International Journal of Molecular Sciences* 12 (6): 3871–87. https://doi.org/10.3390/ijms12063871.

80 Mas-Capdevila, Anna, Joan Teichenne, Cristina Domenech-Coca, Antoni Caimari, Josep M Del Bas, Xavier Escoté, and Anna Crescenti. 2020. "Effect of Hesperidin on Cardiovascular Disease Risk Factors: The Role of Intestinal Microbiota on Hesperidin Bioavailability." *Nutrients* 12 (5): 1488. https://doi.org/10.3390/nu12051488.

81 Man, Mao-Qiang, Bin Yang, and Peter M. Elias. 2019. "Benefits of Hesperidin for Cutaneous Functions." *Evidence-Based Complementary and Alternative Medicine* 2019 (April): 1–19. https://doi.org/10.1155/2019/2676307.

82 Lam, Kit Ying, Anna Pick Kiong Ling, Rhun Yian Koh, Ying Pei Wong, and Yee How Say. 2016. "A Review on Medicinal Properties of Orientin." *Advances in Pharmacological Sciences* 2016: 1–9. https://doi.org/10.1155/2016/4104595.

83 Sunil, Christudas, and Baojun Xu. 2019. "An Insight into the Health-Promoting Effects of Taxifolin (Dihydroquercetin)." *Phytochemistry* 166 (October): 112066. https://doi.org/10.1016/j.phytochem.2019.112066.

84 "Fig. 1. Chemical Structure of Aromadendrin." n.d. ResearchGate. https://www.researchgate.net/figure/Chemical-structure-of-aromadendrin_fig1_51773071#:~:text=Aromadendrin%20is%20reported%20to%20have.

85 Isemura, Mamoru. 2019. "Catechin in Human Health and Disease." *Molecules* 24 (3). https://doi.org/10.3390/molecules24030528.

86 Azubuike-Osu, Sharon O., Ikenna C. Ohanenye, Claus Jacob, Chukwunonso E. C. C. Ejike, and Chibuike C. Udenigwe. n.d. "Beneficial Role of Vitexin and Isovitexin Flavonoids in the Vascular Endothelium and Cardiovascular System." *Current Nutraceuticals* 2 (2): 127–34. https://www.eurekaselect.com/node/187639/article/beneficial-role-of-vitexin-and-isovitexin-flavonoids-in-the-vascular-endothelium-and-cardiovascular-.

87   Rufino, Ana Teresa, Madalena Ribeiro, Cátia Sousa, Fernando Judas, Lígia Salgueiro, Carlos Cavaleiro, and Alexandrina Ferreira Mendes. 2015. "Evaluation of the Anti-Inflammatory, Anti-Catabolic and Pro-Anabolic Effects of E-Caryophyllene, Myrcene and Limonene in a Cell Model of Osteoarthritis." *European Journal of Pharmacology* 750 (March): 141–50. https://doi.org/10.1016/j.ejphar.2015.01.018.

88   Lee, Jeong-Ho, Kicheol Lee, Da Hyun Lee, Soon Young Shin, Yeonjoong Yong, and Young Han Lee. 2015. "Anti-Invasive Effect of β-Myrcene, a Component of the Essential Oil from Pinus Koraiensis Cones, in Metastatic MDA-MB-231 Human Breast Cancer Cells." *Journal of the Korean Society for Applied Biological Chemistry* 58 (4): 563–69. https://doi.org/10.1007/s13765-015-0081-3.

89   Vale, T. Gurgel do, E. Couto Furtado, J. G. Santos, and G. S. B. Viana. 2002. "Central Effects of Citral, Myrcene and Limonene, Constituents of Essential Oil Chemotypes from Lippia Alba (Mill.) N.e. Brown." *Phytomedicine: International Journal of Phytotherapy and Phytopharmacology* 9 (8): 709–14. https://doi.org/10.1078/094471102321621304.

90   Hwang, Eunson, Hien T. T. Ngo, Bom Park, Seul-A Seo, Jung-Eun Yang, and Tae-Hoo Yi. 2017. "Myrcene, an Aromatic Volatile Compound, Ameliorates Human Skin Extrinsic Aging via Regulation of MMPs Production." *The American Journal of Chinese Medicine* 45 (05): 1113–24. https://doi.org/10.1142/s0192415x17500604.

91   Russo, Ethan B. 2011. "Taming THC: Potential Cannabis Synergy and Phytocannabinoid-Terpenoid Entourage Effects." *British Journal of Pharmacology* 163 (7): 1344–64. https://doi.org/10.1111/j.1476-5381.2011.01238.x.

92   Russo, Ethan B. 2008. "Cannabinoids in the Management of Difficult to Treat Pain." *Therapeutics and Clinical Risk Management* 4 (1): 245–59. https://www.ncbi.nlm.nih.gov/pmc/articles/PMC2503660/.

93   "How Specific Terpenes Work on Pain, Inflammation, Anxiety and More." n.d. Treadwell Farms. https://www.treadwellfarms.com/blogs/cbd-education/how-specific-terpenes-work-on-pain-inflammation-anxiety-and-more.

94   Sabogal-Guáqueta, Angélica Maria, Edison Osorio, and Gloria Patricia Cardona-Gómez. 2016. "Linalool Reverses Neuropathological and Behavioral Impairments in Old Triple Transgenic Alzheimer's Mice." *Neuropharmacology* 102 (March): 111–20. https://doi.org/10.1016/j.neuropharm.2015.11.002.

95   Ventola, C Lee. 2015. "The Antibiotic Resistance Crisis: Part 1: Causes and Threats." *P & T : A Peer-Reviewed Journal for Formulary Management* 40 (4): 277–83.

96   Weston-Green, Katrina, Helen Clunas, and Carlos Jimenez Naranjo. 2021. "A Review of the Potential Use of Pinene and Linalool as Terpene-Based Medicines for Brain Health: Discovering Novel Therapeutics in the Flavours and Fragrances of Cannabis." *Frontiers in Psychiatry* 12 (August). https://doi.org/10.3389/fpsyt.2021.583211.

97   Kim, Dae-Seung, Hyun-Ja Lee, Yong-Deok Jeon, Yo-Han Han, Ji-Ye Kee, Hyun-Jeong Kim, Hyun-Ji Shin, et al. 2015. "Alpha-Pinene Exhibits Anti-Inflammatory Activity through the Suppression of MAPKs and the NF-KB Pathway in Mouse Peritoneal Macrophages." *The American Journal of Chinese Medicine* 43 (4): 731–42. https://doi.org/10.1142/S0192415X15500457.

98   Salehi, Bahare, Shashi Upadhyay, Ilkay Erdogan Orhan, Arun Kumar Jugran, Sumali L.D. Jayaweera, Daniel A. Dias, Farukh Sharopov, et al. 2019. "Therapeutic Potential of α- and β-Pinene: A Miracle Gift of Nature." *Biomolecules* 9 (11): 738. https://doi.org/10.3390/biom9110738.

99   Satou, Tadaaki, Hikaru Kasuya, Kazumi Maeda, and Kazuo Koike. 2014. "Daily Inhalation of α-Pinene in Mice: Effects on Behavior and Organ Accumulation." *Phytotherapy Research: PTR* 28 (9): 1284–87. https://doi.org/10.1002/ptr.5105.

100 Satou, Tadaaki, Hikaru Kasuya, Kazumi Maeda, and Kazuo Koike. 2014. "Daily Inhalation of α-Pinene in Mice: Effects on Behavior and Organ Accumulation." *Phytotherapy Research: PTR* 28 (9): 1284–87. https://doi.org/10.1002/ptr.5105.

101 Weston-Green, Katrina, Helen Clunas, and Carlos Jimenez Naranjo. 2021. "A Review of the Potential Use of Pinene and Linalool as Terpene-Based Medicines for Brain Health: Discovering Novel Therapeutics in the Flavours and Fragrances of Cannabis." *Frontiers in Psychiatry* 12 (August). https://doi.org/10.3389/fpsyt.2021.583211

102 Tomko, Andrea M., Erin G. Whynot, Lee D. Ellis, and Denis J. Dupré. 2020. "Anti-Cancer Potential of Cannabinoids, Terpenes, and Flavonoids Present in Cannabis." *Cancers* 12 (7): 1985. https://doi.org/10.3390/cancers12071985.

103 Teow, Sin-Yeang, Kitson Liew, Syed A. Ali, Alan Soo-Beng Khoo, and Suat-Cheng Peh. 2016. "Antibacterial Action of Curcumin against Staphylococcus Aureus: A Brief Review." *Journal of Tropical Medicine* 2016: 1–10. https://doi.org/10.1155/2016/2853045.

104 Lee, Yvonne C. 2012. "Effect and Treatment of Chronic Pain in Inflammatory Arthritis." *Current Rheumatology Reports* 15 (1). https://doi.org/10.1007/s11926-012-0300-4.

105 Chaves, Juliana Siqueira, Paulo César Leal, Luis Pianowisky, and João B. Calixto. 2008. "Pharmacokinetics and Tissue Distribution of the Sesquiterpene Alpha-Humulene in Mice." *Planta Medica* 74 (14): 1678–83. https://doi.org/10.1055/s-0028-1088307.

106 Costa, Celso A R A, Thaís C Cury, Bruna O Cassettari, Regina K Takahira, Jorge C Flório, and Mirtes Costa. 2013. "Citrus Aurantium L. Essential Oil Exhibits Anxiolytic-like Activity Mediated by 5-HT1A-Receptors and Reduces Cholesterol after Repeated Oral Treatment." *BMC Complementary and Alternative Medicine* 13 (1). https://doi.org/10.1186/1472-6882-13-42.

107 Lorigooini, Zahra, Shakiba Nasiri Boroujeni, Mohammad Sayyadi-Shahraki, Mohammad Rahimi-Madiseh, Elham Bijad, and Hossein Amini-khoei. 2021. "Limonene through Attenuation of Neuroinflammation and Nitrite Level Exerts Antidepressant-like Effect on Mouse Model of Maternal Separation Stress." Edited by Elisa Rubino. *Behavioural Neurology* 2021 (January): 1–8. https://doi.org/10.1155/2021/8817309.

108 Sun, Jidong. 2007. "D-Limonene: Safety and Clinical Applications." *Alternative Medicine Review: A Journal of Clinical Therapeutic* 12 (3): 259–64. https://pubmed.ncbi.nlm.nih.gov/18072821/.

109 "Terpene of the Month: Ocimene." 2018. *CeresMED*. August 23, 2018. https://ceresmedvt.com/terpene-of-the-month-ocimene/

110 Pasias, Ioannis N., Dimitris D. Ntakoulas, Kalomoira Raptopoulou, Chrysavgi Gardeli, and Charalampos Proestos. 2021. "Chemical Composition of Essential Oils of Aromatic and Medicinal Herbs Cultivated in Greece—Benefits and Drawbacks." *Foods* 10 (10): 2354. https://doi.org/10.3390/foods10102354.

111 Kim, Cheorl-Ho. 2021. "Anti–SARS-CoV-2 Natural Products as Potentially Therapeutic Agents." *Frontiers in Pharmacology* 12 (May). https://doi.org/10.3389/fphar.2021.590509.

112 D'agostino, Tesse, Frippiat, Machouart, and Debourgogne. 2019. "Essential Oils and Their Natural Active Compounds Presenting Antifungal Properties." *Molecules* 24 (20): 3713. https://doi.org/10.3390/molecules24203713.

113 Turkez, Hasan, Elanur Aydın, Fatime Geyikoglu, and Damla Cetin. 2014. "Genotoxic and Oxidative Damage Potentials in Human Lymphocytes after Exposure to Terpinolene in Vitro." *Cytotechnology* 67 (3): 409–18. https://doi.org/10.1007/s10616-014-9698-z.

114 "Why You Should Know about Terpinolene and Its Benefits." n.d. Www.trulieve.com. https://www.trulieve.com/discover/blog/why-you-should-know-about-terpinolene-and-its-benefits.

115 Aydin, Elanur, Hasan Türkez, and Sener Taşdemir. 2013. "Anticancer and Antioxidant Properties of Terpinolene in Rat Brain Cells." Arhiv Za Higijenu Rada I Toksikologiju 64 (3): 415–24. https://doi.org/10.2478/10004-1254-64-2013-2365.

116 "Cannabinoid." n.d. Weedmaps. https://weedmaps.com/learn/dictionary/cannabinoid.

117 Jikomes, Nick. 2019. "List of Major Cannabinoids in Cannabis and Their Effects." Leafly. April 23, 2019. https://www.leafly.com/news/cannabis-101/list-major-cannabinoids-cannabis-effects.

118 "What Is Cannabigerol (CBG)?" n.d. Verywell Mind. https://www.verywellmind.com/cannabigerol-cbg-uses-and-benefits-5085266.

119 "What Is CBC (Cannabichromene)?" 2017. Leaf Science. May 7, 2017. https://www. leafscience.com/2017/05/07/what-is-cbc-cannabichromene/.

120 Shannon, Scott. 2019. "Cannabidiol in Anxiety and Sleep: A Large Case Series." *The Permanente Journal* 23. https://doi.org/10.7812/tpp/18-041.

121 National Academies of Sciences, Engineering, and Medicine, Health and Medicine Division, Board on Population Health and Public Health Practice, and An Evidence. 2017. "Therapeutic Effects of Cannabis and Cannabinoids." Nih.gov. National Academies Press (US). January 12, 2017. https://www.ncbi.nlm.nih.gov/books/ NBK425767/.

122 "CBN." n.d. Cresco Labs. https://www.crescolabs.com/cannabinoids/ cbn/#:~:text=CBN%20is%20created%20when%20THC.

123 "Cannabicyclol - (CBL) CANNABINOID - Benefits | Effects | Legal Status." n.d. Cannabis Economy. Accessed April 28, 2022. https://canneconomy.com/report/ cannabinoid-report-cbl/.

124 "Cannabinoid Report: CBE." n.d. Cannabis Economy. Accessed April 28, 2022. https:// canneconomy.com/report/cannabinoid-report-cbe/.

125 Nagarkatti, Prakash, Rupal Pandey, Sadiye Amcaoglu Rieder, Venkatesh L Hegde, and Mitzi Nagarkatti. 2009. "Cannabinoids as Novel Anti-Inflammatory Drugs." *Future Medicinal Chemistry* 1 (7): 1333–49. https://doi.org/10.4155/fmc.09.93.

126 Maroon, Joseph, and Jeff Bost. 2018. "Review of the Neurological Benefits of Phytocannabinoids." *Surgical Neurology International* 9 (1): 91. https://doi. org/10.4103/sni.sni_45_18.

127 "What Is THCV and What Are the Benefits of This Cannabinoid?" 2015. Leafly. February 3, 2015. https://www.leafly.com/news/cannabis-101/ what-is-thcv-and-what-are-the-benefits-of-this-cannabinoid.

128 "What Is THCV and What Are the Benefits of This Cannabinoid?" 2015. Leafly. February 3, 2015. https://www.leafly.com/news/cannabis-101/ what-is-thcv-and-what-are-the-benefits-of-this-cannabinoid.

129 "Cannabichromevarin (CBCV)." n.d. Marijuana Doctors | Online Medical Card Directory. https://www.marijuanadoctors.com/weed-101/cannabis-dictionary/ cannabichromevarin-cbcv/.

130 "What Is Cannabigerovarin (CBGV)?" n.d. Marijuana Doctors | Online Medical Card Directory. https://www.marijuanadoctors.com/weed-101/cannabis-dictionary/ cannabigerovarin-cbgv/.

131 New Phase Blends. n.d. "CANNABIGEROL MONOETHYLETHER (CBGM) | New Phase Blends." https://www.newphaseblends.com/cannabigerol-monoethylether-cb-gm/#:~:text=WHAT%20IS%20CANNABIGEROL%20MONOETHYLETHER%20 (CBGM.

132 Evanoff, Anastasia B., Tiffany Quan, Carolyn Dufault, Michael Awad, and Laura Jean Bierut. 2017. "Physicians-In-Training Are Not Prepared to Prescribe Medical Marijuana." *Drug and Alcohol Dependence* 180 (November): 151–55. https://doi.org/10.1016/j.drugalcdep.2017.08.010.

133 "Benefits of CBD with Dr David Allen." n.d. Www.youtube.com. https://www.youtube.com/watch?v=nEsghIeaCOo.

134 "Scientific American Print + Digital Subscription - Copy." n.d. *Scientific American*. https://www.scientificamerican.com/store/subscribe/scientific-american-print1/?utm_source=promotion&utm_medium=sem&utm_campaign=google-adwords&utm_content=text&utm_term=SCA1-US&gclid=EAIaIQobChMItrag_-ya6gIVjsDACh1l1gnyEAAYASAAEgJBmfD_BwE.

135 MD, Peter Grinspoon. 2021. "The Endocannabinoid System: Essential and Mysterious." *Harvard Health*. August 11, 2021. https://www.health.harvard.edu/blog/the-endocannabinoid-system-essential-and-mysterious-202108112569.

136 Scherer, Thomas, and Christoph Buettner. 2009. "The Dysregulation of the Endocannabinoid System in Diabesity—a Tricky Problem." *Journal of Molecular Medicine* 87 (7): 663–68. https://doi.org/10.1007/s00109-009-0459-y.

137 Peres, Fernanda F., Alvaro C. Lima, Jaime E. C. Hallak, José A. Crippa, Regina H. Silva, and Vanessa C. Abílio. 2018. "Cannabidiol as a Promising Strategy to Treat and Prevent Movement Disorders?" *Frontiers in Pharmacology* 9 (May). https://doi.org/10.3389/fphar.2018.00482.

138 De Gregorio, Danilo, Ryan J. McLaughlin, Luca Posa, Rafael Ochoa-Sanchez, Justine Enns, Martha Lopez-Canul, Matthew Aboud, Sabatino Maione, Stefano Comai, and Gabriella Gobbi. 2019. "Cannabidiol Modulates Serotonergic Transmission and Reverses Both Allodynia and Anxiety-like Behavior in a Model of Neuropathic Pain." *PAIN* 160 (1): 136–50. https://doi.org/10.1097/j.pain.0000000000001386.

139 Whyte, L. S., E. Ryberg, N. A. Sims, S. A. Ridge, K. Mackie, P. J. Greasley, R. A. Ross, and M. J. Rogers. 2009. "The Putative Cannabinoid Receptor GPR55 Affects Osteoclast Function in Vitro and Bone Mass in Vivo." *Proceedings of the National Academy of Sciences* 106 (38): 16511–16. https://doi.org/10.1073/pnas.0902743106.

140 Seltzer, Emily S., Andrea K. Watters, Danny MacKenzie, Lauren M. Granat, and Dong Zhang. 2020. "Cannabidiol (CBD) as a Promising Anti-Cancer Drug." *Cancers* 12 (11): 3203. https://doi.org/10.3390/cancers12113203.

141 O'Sullivan, Saoirse Elizabeth. 2016. "An Update on PPAR Activation by Cannabinoids." *British Journal of Pharmacology* 173 (12): 1899–1910. https://doi.org/10.1111/bph.13497.

142 Russo, Ethan B. 2004. "Clinical Endocannabinoid Deficiency (CECD): Can This Concept Explain Therapeutic Benefits of Cannabis in Migraine, Fibromyalgia, Irritable Bowel Syndrome and Other Treatment-Resistant Conditions?" *Neuro Endocrinology Letters* 25 (1-2): 31–39. https://pubmed.ncbi.nlm.nih.gov/15159679/.

143 Loprinzi, Paul D., Liye Zou, and Hong Li. 2019. "The Endocannabinoid System as a Potential Mechanism through Which Exercise Influences Episodic Memory Function." *Brain Sciences* 9 (5): 112. https://doi.org/10.3390/brainsci9050112.

144 Bíró, Tamás, Balázs I. Tóth, György Haskó, Ralf Paus, and Pál Pacher. 2009. "The Endocannabinoid System of the Skin in Health and Disease: Novel Perspectives and Therapeutic Opportunities." *Trends in Pharmacological Sciences* 30 (8): 411–20. https://doi.org/10.1016/j.tips.2009.05.004.

145 "The ECS in Skin." n.d. *Phytecs.* http://www.phytecs.com/tour-the-ecs/the-ecs-in-skin/.

146 Russo, Ethan B. 2016. "Clinical Endocannabinoid Deficiency Reconsidered: Current Research Supports the Theory in Migraine, Fibromyalgia, Irritable Bowel, and Other Treatment-Resistant Syndromes." *Cannabis and Cannabinoid Research* 1 (1): 154–65. https://doi.org/10.1089/can.2016.0009.

147 Russo, Ethan B. 2016. "Clinical Endocannabinoid Deficiency Reconsidered: Current Research Supports the Theory in Migraine, Fibromyalgia, Irritable Bowel, and Other Treatment-Resistant Syndromes." *Cannabis and Cannabinoid Research* 1 (1): 154–65. https://doi.org/10.1089/can.2016.0009.

148 "What Is Endocannabinoid Tone & Why Is It Important?" n.d. Hellomd.com. https://www.hellomd.com/articles/what-is-endocannabinoid-tone-and-why-is-it-important.

149 Meng, Howard, Bradley Johnston, Marina Englesakis, Dwight E. Moulin, and Anuj Bhatia. 2017. "Selective Cannabinoids for Chronic Neuropathic Pain." *Anesthesia & Analgesia* 125 (5): 1638–52. https://doi.org/10.1213/ane.0000000000002110.

150 Hammell, D.C., L.P. Zhang, F. Ma, S.M. Abshire, S.L. McIlwrath, A.L. Stinchcomb, and K.N. Westlund. 2015. "Transdermal Cannabidiol Reduces Inflammation and Pain-Related Behaviours in a Rat Model of Arthritis." *European Journal of Pain* 20 (6): 936–48. https://doi.org/10.1002/ejp.818.

151 Xiong, Wei, Tanxing Cui, Kejun Cheng, Fei Yang, Shao-Rui Chen, Dan Willenbring, Yun Guan, et al. 2012. "Cannabinoids Suppress Inflammatory and Neuropathic Pain by Targeting α3 Glycine Receptors." *The Journal of Experimental Medicine* 209 (6): 1121–34. https://doi.org/10.1084/jem.20120242.

152 Mental Health America. 2016. "Chronic Pain and Mental Health | Mental Health America." Mhanational.org. 2016. https://www.mhanational.org/chronic-pain-and-mental-health.

153 "Introduction to the Endocannabinoid System." n.d. NORML. https://norml.org/marijuana/library/recent-medical-marijuana-research/introduction-to-the-endocannabinoid-system/.

154 "Conant v. Walters, 309 F.3d 629 | Casetext Search + Citator." n.d. Casetext.com. Accessed April 28, 2022. https://casetext.com/case/conant-v-walters.

155 Lynch, Tom, and Amy Price Neff. 2007. "The Effect of Cytochrome P450 Metabolism on Drug Response, Interactions, and Adverse Effects." *American Family Physician* 76 (3): 391–96. https://www.aafp.org/afp/2007/0801/p391.html#:~:text=Because%20 they%20are%20known%20to.

156 "Endocannabinoid Research Group (ERG)." n.d. Nature Index. https://www.natureindex.com/institution-outputs/italy/ endocannabinoid-research-group-erg/521d7052140ba0e335000016#research.

157 Parray, Hilal Ahmad, and Jong Won Yun. 2016. "Cannabidiol Promotes Browning in 3T3-L1 Adipocytes." *Molecular and Cellular Biochemistry* 416 (1-2): 131–39. https:// doi.org/10.1007/s11010-016-2702-5

158 "The US Cannabis Industry Now Supports 321,000 Full-Time Jobs." 2021. Leafly. February 16, 2021. https://www.leafly.com/news/industry/cannabis-jobs-report.

159 CBD Goes Mainstream. 2019. "CBD Goes Mainstream." *Consumer Reports*. April 11, 2019. https://www.consumerreports.org/cbd/cbd-goes-mainstream/.

160 Brenan, Megan. 2019. "14% of Americans Say They Use CBD Products." Gallup. com. Gallup. August 7, 2019. https://news.gallup.com/poll/263147/ameri- cans-say-cbd-products.aspx.

161 "Millennials and Gen Xers Account for over Two-Thirds of U.S. CBD Users, Data Firm Says." n.d. Www.leafreport.com. https://www.leafreport.com/news/millennials- and-gen-xers-account-for-over-two-thirds-of-u-s-cbd-users-data-firm-says-12430.

162 "CBD E-Commerce Sales U.S. 2019-2026." n.d. Statista. Accessed April 28, 2022. https://www.statista.com/statistics/1244901/cbd-e-commerce-sales-us/.

163 Cohen, Koby, and Aviv M. Weinstein. 2018. "Synthetic and Non-Synthetic Cannabinoid Drugs and Their Adverse Effects-A Review from Public Health Perspective." *Frontiers in Public Health* 6 (June). https://doi.org/10.3389/ fpubh.2018.00162.

164 Office of the Commissioner. 2019. "FDA Regulation of Cannabis and Cannabis-Derived Products: Q&A." U.S. Food and Drug Administration. 2019. https://www.fda.gov/news-events/public-health-focus/ fda-regulation-cannabis-and-cannabis-derived-products-including-cannabidiol-cbd.

165 Leweke, F M, D Piomelli, F Pahlisch, D Muhl, C W Gerth, C Hoyer, J Klosterkötter, M Hellmich, and D Koethe. 2012. "Cannabidiol Enhances Anandamide Signaling and Alleviates Psychotic Symptoms of Schizophrenia." *Translational Psychiatry* 2 (3): e94–94. https://doi.org/10.1038/tp.2012.15.

166 Eisenstein, Michael. 2019. "The Reality behind Cannabidiol's Medical Hype." *Nature* 572 (August): S2–4. https://doi.org/10.1038/d41586-019-02524-5.

167 Bergamaschi, Mateus M, Regina Helena Costa Queiroz, Marcos Hortes Nisihara Chagas, Danielle Chaves Gomes de Oliveira, Bruno Spinosa De Martinis, Flávio Kapczinski, João Quevedo, et al. 2011. "Cannabidiol Reduces the Anxiety Induced by Simulated Public Speaking in Treatment-Naïve Social Phobia Patients." *Neuropsychopharmacology* 36 (6): 1219–26. https://doi.org/10.1038/npp.2011.6.

168 Prud'homme, Mélissa, Romulus Cata, and Didier Jutras-Aswad. 2015. "Cannabidiol as an Intervention for Addictive Behaviors: A Systematic Review of the Evidence." *Substance Abuse: Research and Treatment* 9 (January): SART.S25081. https://doi.org/10.4137/sart.s25081

169 Smithburger, Pamela L., Michael A. Zemaitis, and Susan M. Meyer. 2019. "Evaluation of Medical Marijuana Topics in the PharmD Curriculum: A National Survey of Schools and Colleges of Pharmacy." *Currents in Pharmacy Teaching and Learning* 11 (1): 1–9. https://doi.org/10.1016/j.cptl.2018.09.022.

170 "Pharmacists and the Future of Cannabis Medicine." 2020. *Journal of the American Pharmacists Association* 60 (1): 207–11. https://doi.org/10.1016/j.japh.2019.11.007.

171 Zou, Shenglong, and Ujendra Kumar. 2018. "Cannabinoid Receptors and the Endocannabinoid System: Signaling and Function in the Central Nervous System." *International Journal of Molecular Sciences* 19 (3): 833. https://doi.org/10.3390/ijms19030833.

172 "Embracing Feedback: Brands Are Listening to Stakeholder Voices on Racial Injustice." 2020. Porter Novelli. June 12, 2020. https://www.porternovelli.com/intelligence/2020/06/12/embracing-feedback-brands-are-listening-to-stakeholder-voices-on-racial-injustice/.

173 The, Case for Racial, and Equity. n.d. "THE BUSINESS CASE for RACIAL EQUITY a STRATEGY for GROWTH 2018." http://www.nationalcivicleague.org/wp-content/uploads/2018/04/RacialEquityNationalReport-kellogg.pdf.

174 Hudak, John. 2021. "Reversing the War on Drugs: A Five-Point Plan." Brookings. July 7, 2021. https://www.brookings.edu/research/reversing-the-war-on-drugs-a-five-point-plan/.

175 Berg, Larry, and Jackie Berg. 2020. "10 Reasons Why CBD Brands Need to Tap into Multicultural Marketing Now." CBD Marketing Hub. August 11, 2020. https://cbdmarketinghub.com/news/10-reasons-why-cbd-brands-need-to-tap-into-multicultural-marketing-now/.

176 Org, Thecannabisindustry, and Policycouncil. 2020. "Learn More about NCIA's Policy Council ENVIRONMENTAL SUSTAINABILITY in the CANNABIS INDUSTRY IMPACTS, BEST MANAGEMENT PRACTICES, and POLICY CONSIDERATIONS." https://thecannabisindustry.org/wp-content/uploads/2020/11/NCIA-Environmental-Policy-BMP-October-17-final.pdf.

Made in the USA
Las Vegas, NV
15 February 2023

67578442R00131